From Scattered to Centered

Understanding and Transforming
The ADHD Brain

By Alicia R. Maher, MD

Edited by

Susan Macaulay and Suzanna Gratz

Published by
PESI Publishing & Media
PESI, Inc
3839 White Ave
Eau Claire, WI 54703

Cover Design: Amy Rubenzer
Layout Design: Bookmasters
Edited By: Susan Maculay & Suzanna Gratz

Printed in the United States of America

ISBN: 978-1-937661-63-2

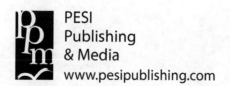

PESI
Publishing
& Media
www.pesipublishing.com

To Mirko, thank you for the inspiration, support and encouragement that made this book possible and for the abundant joy in which we live.

And thank you to my mother, Elaine, for providing the foundation for so much of this content.

Table of Contents

Introduction

WE'RE ALL IN THE SAME BOAT

"If only they knew," I often think to myself as I listen to my patients describe their symptoms of restlessness and distraction. . ."if only they knew how alike we are!"

In my years as a physician and practicing psychiatrist, innumerable clients have recounted stories which could just as easily be my own. They feel like they're going to explode when they're asked to sit still. They can't maintain focus on one thought for more than a few seconds. The rest of the world seems to move at a snail's pace. Oh yes. I've been in their shoes—a lone soldier marching to the beat of a different drummer. It's been like that since I was young.

"Alicia, sit still!" Ms.Drake, my first grade teacher, would admonish. She might as well have asked me to fly–that anyone could sit in one place for more than a few minutes was inconceivable to me. I marveled at my classmates who could be relatively still for hours on end when there was a whole world to explore and so many things to do. What was wrong with them? After having my desk put in the hallway for the hundredth time, it occurred to me that it wasn't the other kids that were different–it was me.

Not that I blame Ms. Drake for my repeated banishments. After all, she had lessons to teach, and my disrupting the class with nonstop talking and fidgeting made her task next to impossible.

Over and over, I was reprimanded and told what to do and what not to do. But no matter what punishments I faced, I just couldn't behave myself. I wanted to. I really did. I wanted to pay attention, to listen and play nicely; I just couldn't figure out how. Some unknown force drove me to misbehave and blurt out the first thought that came to my head before I even realized what was happening. It was hell all around. I was as frustrated by my inability to control myself as the adults around me were by my seemingly endless capacity for disobedience and mischief.

Day after day, my mother tried to drill into me organizational skills such as making lists and schedules, and keeping track of objects. Night after night, she tirelessly dragged me through my homework. Unfortunately, though her homework assistance helped me flourish academically, my failure with lists and schedules locked her into the role of taskmaster for most of my childhood.

MEDICINE? YOU MUST BE KIDDING!

Though a career in medicine may not seem like the logical outcome of this story, my fascination with human physiology compelled me to enter medical school to pursue a career as a surgeon. After high school, I was accepted into a six-year program that combined college and medical school. Luckily, the early years of this program were highly structured. I didn't have to keep track of life's little details, and I was far too busy studying to get into trouble—with a few notable exceptions!

On cross-state road trips in my student days, I usually drove with the "pedal to the metal," oblivious of the speedometer and the speed limits. I cringe today when I think of the danger in which I put others and myself with my recklessness. Although most of my journeys were without incident, one day I sped by a radar trap, prompting the officer who manned it to give chase. Unable to keep up with me because he was confined to 75 mph, he radioed ahead and about a half an hour later I saw flashing lights in the rearview mirror. By this time I was cruising at 119 mph in a 55 mph zone, and, though I was too distracted to notice, I had been part of a high-speed police pursuit. I was arrested and spent a day in jail.

Such incidents were so typical in my life that I was hardly bothered, though I remembered feeling inconvenienced by having to study frantically for an exam while behind bars! Thankfully I passed the test AND learned to be more diligent in monitoring my speed while driving.

I managed reasonably well and made good grades during the structured basic science years of medical school. But as we transitioned into clinical work, the lack of structure left me feeling overwhelmed and inadequate. My peers eagerly donned white coats and seemed intuitively to know how to talk to patients and manage their diverse hospital work, while I desperately searched for something or someone to guide me and keep me on task.

My initial goal had been to become a surgeon, but I was quickly drawn into the world of psychiatry. Whereas medical treatment patched up a patient's body, psychiatric treatment seemed to delve deeper into the how and why a person came to need help in the first place. I saw that people could actually use their brains to dramatically change their lives for the better. Ironically, despite my passion for the subject, the actual practice of psychiatry drove me crazy! As patients told me their stories, I became buried in the avalanche of details, unable to focus or determine what was relevant among the flurry of information. Luckily, this would soon change.

During the first year studying psychiatry, interns mainly learn by following around doctors more experienced in the field and observing how they diagnose and manage patients. Despite my knowledge and experience, I seemed unable to cope with the classes, the schedule, the curriculum—you name it, I had a problem with it. My professors constantly chided me over one issue or another. But the benefit of working with psychiatrists was that they could easily diagnose the underlying cause of the daily struggle that overwhelmed me. They pointed out my lack of organization, and the fact that I was able to handle far less than my peers despite having fewer tasks overall. They forced me to focus, prioritize, and organize, but often their efforts failed. Finally, in somewhat of an intervention, several of my professors got together and confronted me with a list of their various complaints.

"We believe," they said, "that you have Attention Deficit Hyperactivity Disorder."

THE "SHOCKING" TRUTH

Once the words were spoken, I was shocked that the diagnosis hadn't occurred to me before. But as I looked back over my life, it seemed so obvious. Upon reading further about the illness, I realized mine was a classic case. All of a sudden, my suspicion that I wasn't a "bad kid" was confirmed. Everyone had been right: there was something different about me, but now I knew why.

My professors didn't tell me to get treatment, but they made it clear that I had better do something–they were done picking up the slack for me. I had no intention of letting go of my dream of becoming a psychiatrist, so it wasn't long before I took concrete steps that would change my life, and allow me to successfully complete my medical training.

Because you're reading this book, I'm assuming you and I have a lot in common, just like I have a lot in common with many of my patients. You're looking for answers, or at least guidance, about how to fit into a world that seems to be mired in structure and moving in slow motion. Believe me, I know the day-to-day frustration you feel when life bombards you with minutia and timetables, when your family and colleagues roll their eyes and tease (or complain) about your inability to complete simple tasks, and when all you want to do is be normal.

I wrote this book with the hope that my journey, with all its adventures (and misadventures!), might provide some insight into the challenging, yet manageable world of ADHD. What is this syndrome with which up to 10 percent of children and about 5 percent of adults are diagnosed? Are you one of them? And most important, is there a cure?

While there are definite neurophysiological causes and well-defined symptoms of ADHD, diagnosis can be difficult. When working with children, one has to determine whether the behavior is that of a kid just being a kid, or whether it's something more. In adults, especially in today's media-centric, instant gratification-based world, it's sometimes difficult to differentiate between the symptoms of ADHD and the results of living in a fast-paced society. In the chapters that follow, we'll delve deeper into the most common symptoms of ADHD and clarify the differences between it and the perils of living a hectic, modern lifestyle.

The good news is that, in my professional opinion and judging from my own personal experience and those of many of my patients, there are definitely ways to manage the symptoms of ADHD–both through medication and alternative treatments such as yoga and meditation. In my own life, treatment has led me to become the fully competent, in control, confident person I have wanted to be ever since those elementary school days when I spent a great deal of time at a desk in the hall instead of in the classroom. It's sometimes hard to accept, after all of my years of struggle, that life can actually be lived with relative ease. In fact, the people that currently surround me find it difficult to believe that I even carry this diagnosis.

You Too Can Rewire Your Brain

In this book you'll find information about a variety of treatments and key brain-changing exercises that address each of the symptoms of ADHD.

Thanks to modern discoveries in neuroscience, we now know that we can rewire our brains on a structural level, and change the way they function. As you read this book, I encourage you to go through the exercises and try those that you think might be helpful. Do this with as many exercises as you need–you can even do more than one at a time. The key to making change in the brain is to do the exercises consistently (i.e. daily), and over the long term (i.e. months and years, not days and weeks).

If you apply a particular exercise consistently for 30 days, you will train your brain to function differently in that particular area. Though it varies, 30 days is the average amount of time required to create noticeable change. However, if there are gaps in those 30 days, (i.e. if the practice isn't done daily), more time may be necessary.

Please keep in mind that no part of this book is meant to replace evaluation or treatment by a professional. Nor are all of the treatments described in this book recognized as standards of care or FDA approved. Rather, this book is meant to get you started on the path towards understanding issues you may experience and expand your awareness of how to manage them.

One last thought before we get started on our exploration of ADHD: while I've had great success in keeping my ADHD at bay, there are amazing qualities about my life that are likely there because of ADHD. It many ways, ADHD is a gift as well as a curse.

For most of us, it's a matter of balancing that extra zing with a little more structure so we're able to enjoy our magical lives without the constant need for a clean-up crew. I was able to find that balance, and I'm confident that, if you take the necessary steps, you will too. The brain is powerful. The truth is that you can use that power to take control and create the life you desire.

Alicia R. Maher, M.D.

Overview

Do YOU Have ADHD?

I've lost count of the number of times I've heard the question: "Do I have ADHD, Dr. Maher?" I've been asked this so frequently, perhaps because many of the symptoms of attention deficit disorders are also seen in "normal" individuals. In this modern world of endless distractions, someone without an attention disorder may have many of the same symptoms as someone who has one. This chapter will shed some light on what ADHD is, and how it's diagnosed.

Different forms of attention disorders, hyperactivity, and impulsivity are often grouped under the catchall label Attention Deficit Disorder, or ADD, as it is commonly known. Usually, the acronym ADD refers to attention deficit disorder, while ADHD stands for Attention Deficit Hyperactivity Disorder. To be diagnosed with ADHD, a person must have attention deficit disorder accompanied by hyperactive and/or impulsive behaviors. Either set of symptoms/behaviors may predominate, or be present in equal measure, but both conditions must be present. For consistency, I will use the acronym ADHD to mean either condition; when referring only to ADD, I will make the distinction. Also, I will use the terms "ADHDers" and "non-ADHDers" respectively in reference to those with and without the condition.

Everyone is different and circumstances vary, so this overview (and in fact this whole book), is not meant to replace diagnosis and treatment by a professional. If you suspect that you, or someone you care about, has ADD or ADHD, I highly recommend that you seek professional help. I repeat this advice many times in this book because it's important: self-diagnosis and self-treatment are neither reliable nor desirable.

Knowledge and information are useful. They can help one sort out a disorder that to many people is a confusing puzzle with all kinds of pieces that don't seem to fit. This book will provide you with the tools you need to better understand your condition, and empower you to discuss it intelligently with a trained professional if need be. That's why I'd like to begin with a short quiz that introduces the main symptoms of ADHD.

Like most "diagnostic" quizzes, this is designed to help you consider your behavior, not to diagnose your condition. Still, the quiz is a quick and easy way to give you an indication of whether you may have ADHD. If the quiz results show that you may have ADHD, I strongly recommend that you make an appointment with a qualified professional who is equipped to make a definitive diagnosis.

Here's how to take the quiz: answer "true" to a statement only if the behavior or characteristic is an enduring part of your personality, not just the way you may have behaved recently, or on occasion when you may have been stressed. If you answer "true" to a statement, that particular behavior should be severe enough to have caused problems for you in your relationships or functioning during the last six months.

ADHD Behavior/Symptoms Quiz

Part I.

1. When someone tells me how to do something, I listen to get an overall picture, but I get overwhelmed or anxious if they give too many details.

   a) True

   b) False

2. I find it virtually impossible to complete a task or project that doesn't interest me. I constantly take breaks to do other things.

   a) True

   b) False

3. For the most part, I cannot maintain one train of thought. My mind is full of all kinds of different ideas.

   a) True

   b) False

4. I tend to avoid things that require me to maintain focus or concentration for long periods of time such as books with involved plots or complicated puzzles.

   a) True

   b) False

5. I have many partially completed projects.

   a) True

   b) False

6. It is not uncommon for me (and/or others), to find many careless mistakes in my work.

   a) True

   b) False

7. No one would mistake my house for that of Martha Stewart (i.e.: I am definitely NOT organized!)

   a) True

   b) False

8. I constantly misplace everyday items such as keys, wallets, etc.

   a) True

   b) False

9. I often forget to bring things that are key to completing a task.

   a) True

   b) False

Part II.

10. People complain that I'm not listening to them, even when I think I am.

   a) True

   b) False

11. I like to talk more than listen.

   a) True

   b) False

12. I feel good when I'm stimulated and active.

   a) True

   b) False

13. I quickly become depressed when not engaged in activity.

   c) True

   d) False

14. I have trouble doing activities that require sitting still, such as watching a movie.

   a) True

   b) False

15. Waiting in line or sitting in traffic seems like an annoyance to others, but it feels like torture to me!

    a) True

    b) False

16. I feel an underlying sense that I need to be doing something, but I'm often not sure what it is.

    a) True

    b) False

17. No one would ever describe me as a quiet person.

    a) True

    b) False

18. I find it difficult to follow rules such as speed limits.

    a) True

    b) False

19. I often interrupt others when they're speaking because I have the gist of what they're saying before they finish saying it.

    a) True

    b) False

20. In meetings, I feel compelled to blurt out whatever comes to mind, even if someone else is still talking.

    a) True

    b) False

EVALUATING YOUR QUIZ RESULTS

Add up the number of "true" statements.

> Part I. Six or more 'true' statements are indicative of issues with attention deficit and/or inattention.
>
> Part II. Six or more 'true' statements are indicative of issues with impulsivity and/or hyperactivity.

If you answered 'true' to six or more statements in both Part I and II, this indicates both deficits in attention and issues with hyperactivity.

If you have experienced these behaviors and/or symptoms since be-fore the age of seven, you may have Attention Deficit Disorder or Attention Deficit Hyperactivity Disorder. Remember: taking a short quiz such as this is not sufficient to make a diagnosis! If you suspect you have ADD or ADHD, I strongly urge you to talk to a qualified professional, to find out how to get properly assessed and diagnosed.

Let me make another cautionary note. Many of us in "modern" societies experience some of these symptoms simply by virtue of the way we choose to live: in fast-paced, information-packed, highly stimulating environments. Others may experience some of these symptoms as a result of the life stage in which they find themselves. For example, perimenopausal and menopausal women often complain of forgetfulness and lack of focus, as do many elderly folk of both genders.

Whether your symptoms are caused by genetics, electronics, or your life stage, I will help you put the puzzle pieces together and better understand the causes that may lie behind the behaviors and symptoms you identified in the quiz. I will also suggest concrete steps you can take to train your brain to work in a way that is more centered and effective.

To help you focus on the bits of the puzzle that might be of particular interest to you, I've created the following reference chart to help you navigate quickly and easily to personally relevant chapters.

Chart 1 Chapter Contents

Chapter	Topic	Quiz Statement #
	Overview	All
1	Focus	1, 2, 3
2	Follow Through	4, 5, 6
3	Disorganization	7, 8, 9
4	Social Issues	10, 11
5	Emotional Reactivity	12, 13
6	Inner Restlessness	14, 15, 16
7	Impulsivity	17, 18, 19, 20

As I discuss the various symptoms of Attention Deficit Hyperactivity Disorder, I'll also share research suggesting that modern technology may be altering our brains to make many of us behave in 'ADHD-like' ways.

What Causes ADHD and Its Symptoms?

ADHD is a biological illness, the exact cause of which is as yet undetermined; although it is known that ADHD brains function differently than "normal" brains. Specifically, they seem to process neurochemicals in unusual ways.

Neurochemicals facilitate the communication between our brain cells, which in turn give instructions to our body to enable it to function properly and complete tasks. The neurons in ADHD brains, however, seem to fail to appropriately process these neurochemicals. This may explain why high doses of neurochemicals in certain medications produce the opposite effects in AD-HDers than they do in non-ADHDers. For example, stimulants—the most common form of treatment for ADHD—should stimulate, as their name implies. However, administering stimulants to inattentive, hyperactive ADHDers causes them to gain focus, slow down and become calmer. Solid existing research demonstrates a relationship between ADHD and altered neurochemical processing, but more is needed to fully explain how it impacts brain functions.

Though the processes associated with it are presently not fully understood, one thing is certain, ADHD is a biological, *not* a psychological illness. It is caused by biological factors related to brain functioning that are beyond an ADHDer's control, not to psychological or emotional issues.

Until relatively recently, ADHD was thought to be strictly a childhood disorder. Now we know that people don't "grow out of it." Although some symptoms may change and/or lessen substantially with time, it's estimated at least two-thirds of ADHD kids continue to suffer its effects as adults, and only about 20 percent of adults who have ADHD are diagnosed and treated.

This book focuses on the challenges associated with ADHD in adults. However, ADHD does not develop in adulthood. To be diagnosed with ADHD, even as an adult, one must have experienced ADHD symptoms before the age of seven. That makes diagnosis challenging in adulthood.

What ADHD 'Looks' Like in 'Real' People

Before we explore the symptoms and behaviors associated with ADHD in more detail, I would like to share some examples of the types of cases I see in my psychiatric practice (they are composites for the most part, and the names are fictional):

Tom

Tom has struggled with feeling "different" for as long as he can remember. He often got in trouble for talking out of turn and not following directions as a child. Tom's teachers suggested to his parents that Tom might have ADHD, but he wasn't privy to those conversations. Tom's parents didn't believe ADHD was an illness. They felt such a label would simply provide an excuse for Tom's bad behavior. As a result, Tom spent his childhood feeling bad about himself. He had no answer when people asked: "What is wrong with you?" "Why can't you get it together?" When Tom was finally diagnosed with ADHD as an adult, he was relieved. For Tom, and others like him, knowing there is a biological cause to their behavior is a huge comfort. Once he was diagnosed, Tom was finally able to stop blaming himself and fighting his natural tendencies.

Jim

Jim wasn't diagnosed with ADHD as a child either—but for a different reason. Jim's parents thought he might have ADHD, but they dismissed the possibility when they noticed he could focus for hours on end when he did things he enjoyed, such as playing video games. They decided Jim was just lazy, and only wanted to do things he liked. This is a common barrier in diagnosing ADHD. Activities that capture their interest and provide instant feedback can keep ADHDers engaged for long periods. However, repetitive and uninteresting tasks, which require them to draw on the brain in a different way, are problematic. To make a proper diagnosis, it's important to explore how the individual behaves in a diversity of circumstances and environments. Jim's parents would have done him a big favor by taking him to see a professional with the skills to properly assess his behavior.

Jill and David

Jill's story differs greatly from those of Tom and Jim. Although girls are statistically less likely to suffer ADHD than boys, Jill's parents had her diagnosed and on medication from a young age. Her medications helped her perform adequately in school, but she hated being "abnormal" and often resisted taking them. In high school, she even gave her "meds" away to friends who enjoyed the "high" they got from taking them. This further confirmed to Jill how different she was: the medications didn't make her high, they slowed her down! She often wished she could be like her friends and also get a "buzz."

Jill's friend David also seemed to have ADHD. He was always distracted, never paid full attention to conversations and texted constantly. Taking Jill's medications gave David the energy he needed to complete research papers. But the stimulants also made him more hyper and scattered. Though many suspected his listening and focus issues to be ADHD-related, it was obvious to Jill they were more likely just bad habits. He didn't experience the same things she did, and her medications certainly didn't slow him down the way they did her.

Sylvia

Sylvia wasn't diagnosed with ADHD until adulthood. As a child, she had trouble following what was said. She lived in a daydream, rarely paying attention to what was going on around her. She was often restless, yet so shy she spoke infrequently and never caused trouble. Like many young girls whose symptoms are predominantly associated with inattentiveness (she was not hyperactive), her struggle went largely unnoticed. People just assumed she wasn't very bright. It wasn't until she had a daughter of her own, and her daughter was tested for ADHD, that Sylvia's ADHD was discovered. She recognized, in her daughter's test results, many of the symptoms with which she herself had suffered as a child. She was then tested, and finally started getting the treatment she needed. It was like a second chance at life. She realized she wasn't "stupid" or inept, but rather had a common illness she could manage with the right medication.

Josh

Josh was a troublemaker in his youth, and his issues became increasingly apparent as he grew older. He was the class clown, and his impulsive actions and words often got him into hot water. When ADHD was suspected, Josh was given medication, with disastrous results. The stimulants he took only made his agitation and impulsivity worse. What happened? Josh came from a difficult background, and lacked social skills due to the environment in which he was raised. Furthermore, he had experienced severe head trauma as a child. The head injury had damaged the part of the brain that would have given him the ability to anticipate the results of his actions and refrain from doing those with adverse consequences. The combination of not having the skills to choose the proper actions, coupled with the inability to control himself, made it look like Josh had ADHD. However, because he did not have ADHD, his brain became stimulated when he took stimulants, thus making his issues worse. People with head injuries may have ADHD-like behaviors and symptoms, however, as the cause is different, so too must be the treatment.

DIAGNOSING ADHD

So how did Tom, Jim, Jill, and Sylvia get diagnosed with ADHD? Diverse tools are used in the diagnostic process. When one is diagnosed in childhood, as Jill was, the process can be relatively straightforward. The child must exhibit a certain number of ADHD symptoms/behaviors (see the list below), over an extended period of time of at least 6 months. But making a diagnosis is more complex than simply ticking off items on a list, just as it's more involved than completing the 20-question quiz in this overview.

Parents, teachers and/or trained professionals should observe the child's behavior in multiple environments and circumstances, and document their observations. These observations must then be evaluated to determine exactly which symptoms the child has. Additionally, a thorough medical history should be taken to eliminate other potential causes such as brain injury, psychological problems or other factors of the aberrant behavior.

In adults, like Tom and Jim, things may be a little trickier. To make a correct diagnosis, a doctor must have a clear picture of the individual's childhood behaviors before the age of seven. In the case of the composite examples above, Tom would have had to remember his own childhood behavior—not an easy task after 20, 30 or even 40 years! Jim had an easier go of it–he asked his parents, though they too found it hard to remember that far back.

Knowing an individual was symptomatic as a child can help in making an adulthood diagnosis of ADHD. However, such a diagnosis does not necessarily mean the existing adulthood symptoms are sufficient to warrant treatment. Several written tests have been developed to help diagnose ADHD in adults. Unfortunately, the validity of these tests has not yet been rigorously proven. That's why adulthood diagnoses are still generally made by professionals who talk to the patient extensively, consider a multitude of factors, and carefully evaluate all diagnostic possibilities.

Doctors try to determine which symptoms were present when the patient was a child, what the current problem is, and whether the existing symptoms are due to ADHD, or to other causes. To complicate matters further, there are particular ways in which ADHD symptoms change as one ages. As we discuss the symptoms below and throughout the book, we'll explore what ADHD behaviors look like in children, as well as how they manifest differently in adults.

What about Jill's friend David, who was clearly inattentive and easily distracted, but whose reaction to Jill's medications made it obvious he did not have ADHD?

ADHD-like symptoms may be present in anyone at any given time. However, the parameters for distinguishing those who have ADHD from those who do not are clearly defined:

- The individual must exhibit at least six symptoms of inattention, hyperactivity/impulsivity, or both, for at least six months.

- The symptoms must impact the individual in critical life areas such as relationships and work.
- The symptoms must not be caused by another mental or physical condition (such as a difficult upbringing or a brain injury), bad habits with respect to the use of technology, or other similar factors.

ATTENTION DEFICIT/INATTENTION SYMPTOMS (ADD)

So, what are the symptoms of ADD and ADHD? Let's start with those found in children. As this disorder was first diagnosed in children, the diagnostic criteria are more obvious. To be diagnosed with attention deficit disorder (ADD), a child must have exhibited at least six symptoms of attention deficit/inattention for a minimum of six months; the symptoms must have started before the age of seven.

In children, inattention has several facets: lack of attention to detail, inability to maintain focus, and difficulty completing tasks. ADD children also tend to be easily distracted, make careless mistakes and regularly forget things. Children with ADD often appear inattentive, and rarely pay attention to what they are told. They seem to devote just enough energy to get the gist of what you say, and then tune out additional details. Even when they are attentive, it is difficult for them to maintain their focus for longer than a few minutes. While 10 minutes might seem like a short time for a "normal" child, for example, it is an absolute eternity to an ADD child who is not engaged in an activity he or she does not find mentally or physically stimulating.

ADD children are great at beginnings. They're likely to start several tasks, but tend to be off to the next thing before completing what they have begun. They are like honey bees, buzzing from one flower to the next. While on the flower, they focus for a short time on the task at hand, but they're off to the next bloom in the blink of an eye! They also tend to avoid activities requiring sustained focus, such as problem solving and math. When they do put in effort, they tend to give up quickly if they find a task too challenging.

Compounding their inability to focus is the fact that ADD children are easily distracted. This is another reason they don't seem to be listening when spoken to. It may also contribute to their tendency to make careless mistakes, such as not dotting i's or crossing t's. They know how to do it, but don't notice they aren't doing it correctly. They have difficulty organizing their time and belongings, and seem always to either forget or lose important items such as pieces of clothing, school books, homework, lunch boxes, and the like. A general state of forgetfulness is a common characteristic of a child with ADD.

Hyperactivity Symptoms (The "H" In ADHD)

The hyperactive symptom spectrum includes those of both hyperactivity and impulsivity. As with the symptoms of inattention, a child must have displayed them consistently over time to be diagnosed hyperactive. The child would need to exhibit at least six of the symptoms for at least six months, and again, the behaviors need to have been evident before the age of seven. The symptoms and behaviors associated with hyperactivity and impulsivity are usually more easily observed than those associated with inattentiveness. They include fidgeting, inability to sit still for even short intervals, and constantly being on the move–everywhere, all the time!

Hyperactive/impulsive children are often noisy; speaking loudly, creating a lot of sound by banging, clanging, and hammering anything and everything within reach. They rarely notice the cacophony they've generated, nor do they know it's excessive. Hyperactive children almost never play quietly, unless they are engrossed in a stimulating activity they enjoy, such as video gaming.

Some people worry the exuberance of childhood might be misinterpreted as hyperactivity, but there is a clear difference. The behavior of hyperactive children is several orders of magnitude above exuberant. Moreover, the increased energy level has a definite "edginess" to it–in fact, it would be more accurately described as "agitated" rather than "exuberant." A general sense of restlessness generally permeates the space around an ADHD child. It's almost like a highly charged electrical field surrounds them.

Parents often say they feel as if their ADHD child is driven by a motor with more energy than the child herself actually wants to have. She is like an unwilling Energizer Bunny[1] that's been wound up: she simply cannot stop until her batteries run out. Unfortunately, those batteries seem to keep on going *forever*!

Hyperactive/impulsive children know they should not blurt out answers or talk in class, but feel helpless to stop from doing so. It seems utterly impossible to the child to patiently wait his turn, whether in line for something, or

---

[1] 1994 Star War Energizer Bunny commercial http://www.youtube.com/watch?v=QxafIhYFOr0

simply to speak. Unable to wait, they "jump the queue" and interrupt others mid-thought or mid-sentence.

Children may exhibit symptoms of either inattention or hyperactivity/impulsivity, or both. When evaluating behaviors such as these for a diagnosis, it's important to remember the symptoms must be severe enough to impair the individual's ability to function normally. This is usually quite obvious in children as it is frequently reflected in their academic performance. In adulthood, ADHD challenges occur primarily in an individual's ability to maintain healthy relationships and gainful employment.

Attention Deficit (Inattention) Symptoms/Behaviors

Disregards/ignores details

Seems not to listen

Avoids sustained mental effort

Is easily distracted

Fails to finish tasks

Makes careless mistakes

Unable to organize self and/or environment

Forgets needed items

Loses things frequently

Hyperactivity/Impulsivity Symptoms/Behaviors

Fidgets

Is always restless

Leaves seat at inappropriate times

Speaks loudly

Talks excessively

Makes lots of noise

Seems motor-driven/"wound-up"

Unable to wait for his/her turn

Blurts out answers

Interrupts often

THE SEVEN ADULT SYMPTOMS OF ADHD

While reading through the description above, you may have already recognized childhood symptoms of ADHD sometimes observed in adults. However, due to the altered circumstances of adult life, as well as age-induced changes in the brain, many of these symptoms manifest differently in adulthood. I've divided the adult symptoms into seven types, each of which has a chapter of its own.

As this book is also written for those who experience ADHD-like symptoms as a result of our fast-paced, modern lifestyle, I'll also refer to research suggesting how these symptoms may develop, particularly with respect to the use of technology. Though much research remains to be done in this area, emerging theories and discoveries are thought provoking.

The seven symptoms exhibited by adult ADHDers (and those who behave similarly for other reasons) are:

1. Decreased focus
2. Lack of follow-through
3. Disorganization
4. Social issues
5. Emotional reactivity
6. Inner restlessness
7. Impulsivity

Each of the following seven chapters explains and explores one of the symptoms in more detail. Let's get going!

CHAPTER 1

Decreased Focus

How Lack of Focus Manifests in Adult ADHDers

As we saw in the overview, lack of focus is readily observable in ADHD children. They often appear not to pay attention to anything you tell them. They seem to devote just enough energy to get the gist of what you're saying, and then tune out additional details you try to share. Even when they do pay attention, it is often difficult for them to maintain their focus for more than a few minutes.

Similarly, adult ADHDers have a hard time sustaining attention for extended periods. However, their inability to focus may not be as obvious as the adult workday offers plenty of opportunities to switch tasks, whereas children are expected to focus on one subject at a time in school. Both ADHD children and adults may fly from one thing to another. However, the behavior may be less obvious and less problematic in adults because they can choose the breadth of their activities, whereas children are expected to stay on task, particularly at school.

Lack of focus also contributes to forgetfulness in ADHDers because they have difficulty focusing on details they receive in the moment; this explains in part why both ADHD children and adults find it challenging to recall details after the fact. However, ADHD children and adults differ in this respect: a child may simply be oblivious to detail, where adults may be aware of details to which they should attend, but are unable to do so, perhaps as a subconscious strategy to avoid being overwhelmed by them. Adult ADHD sufferers demonstrate a general inability to pay close attention to details. They do most things in a haphazard or sloppy manner in all areas of their lives, from family life and relationships to study and work activities.

Not everyone who lacks focus has ADHD, however. We all (ADHDer or not) occasionally suffer from a lack of focus. The causes are diverse; they include stress, illness, phase of life, and trying to do too much with too little for too long. The latter is a particularly big problem in this day and age. We simply try to do too many things at the same time—we call it "multitasking."

The term "multitasking" originated in the computer engineering industry in the 1960s. It refers to the ability of a microprocessor's apparent ability to perform several tasks simultaneously. In fact, even computers, despite their amazing technology, are unable to multitask. They actually process information in sequence, but do it so quickly it appears to happen simultaneously. Interestingly, the word "multitask" does not generate a spelling error message in Microsoft Word®, so deeply has it become ingrained in modern language, this, despite the fact that it was virtually unknown as a human activity, as opposed to a computer processing capability, before 1998.[2]

Drive, talk on the phone, manage the kids in the back seat, listen to an audio book, think about what we should be doing next—the lists (and there may be several of them!) go on and on. In one workplace study, researchers found nine out of 10 employees multitasked during conference calls. This included working on other projects, reading email, eating, making phone calls, going to the restroom, and even surfing pornographic Internet sites.[3]

While multitasking may be applauded, and even rewarded, especially in the workplace, it's really not good for us, for a number of different reasons. By trying to do too many things at once, we may end up doing all of them poorly instead of any of them well. Likewise, by taking in too many stimuli at once, we are less able to pay full attention to any one stimulus. The epidemic of multitasking may be contributing to what appears to be an epidemic of ADHD.

If there is learning involved in any of the tasks we do simultaneously, we may be less able to learn effectively, and thus have to "relearn" over and over again. When we multitask, we use different brain systems to lay down memory, and though we may be able to remember the basics of information we receive when we're distracted, our memory is less flexible. This means that while we may be able to repeat back what was said to us, we won't be able to use the knowledge in a meaningful way, and, instead of saving time, we end up wasting time because we must relearn the things we didn't learn properly in the first place![4]

---

[2] *Human multitasking*, Wikipedia, http://en.wikipedia.org/wiki/Human_multitasking
[3] A Different Optic, February 2005, Bloomfield Associates, LLC
[4] *Multi-tasking Adversely Affects Brain's Learning*, Science Daily, July 26, 2006. http://www.sciencedaily.com/releases/2006/07/060726083302.htm

What lies behind lack of focus, and what can be done to manage it? Let's dive in head first (pun definitely intended!) with a look at how the brain works, and how its functioning fits into the ADHD puzzle.

OUR UNDECIDED BRAINS

One of the most interesting characteristics of the brain is that it's wired to 1) make us want to repeat things that feel good, and 2) feel good when we experience new things. That the brain creates these opposing reactions is one of the drivers of some ADHD behaviors, including ADHDers' difficulties with focus.

Let's look at the example of substance abuse to see how the brain causes individuals to repeat "enjoyable" behaviors. We don't abuse or become "addicted" to a substance (and/or behavior, routine, activity, feeling, experience, etc.) because it feels good—although it likely may, initially. Rather, over the long term, it becomes "addictive" because it causes a chemical called *dopamine* "the feel good chemical" to be released in the *nucleus accumbens* (a primitive area of the brain). Over time, continued dopamine release form a learning pathway in the brain. Then, when we do things associated with this action, small amounts of dopamine are released into the learning pathway and thus the brain fosters these dopamine-induced hits of pleasure.

Our "cravings" are caused by the anticipation of the dopamine release in the learning pathway. So, when an 'addict' is neurologically stimulated through their physical senses, a dopamine release pushes them to acquire the experience again. This is the reason why, for some people, the "Just Say No!" advertising campaigns—showing drug paraphernalia though accompanied by a negative command—were unsuccessful. Just the sight of the equipment used to take the drugs can set off neurological cravings, causing 'addicts' to seek out the very experiences the campaigns try to get them to abandon!

CHEAP THRILLS AND THE ADHD BRAIN

Just like some chemical processes in the brain make us want to keep doing "known" things that we enjoy, other chemical processes make us want to 1) do ever-increasing amounts of the same activity, 2) do more intense versions of the same activity and/or 3) do things in the same vein, but that are also somehow new, different and exciting. Why? Because all of them also release dopamine into the brain.

Imagine for a moment that you are learning to cook, and you have just been introduced to spices other than salt and pepper. Your recipe calls for a pinch of basil. You put in the pinch that's required and the dish is delicious, so delicious in fact, that the next time you make it, you put in two pinches, because, you think to yourself: "If one pinch is so tasty, two pinches must be twice as nice." Next time it's three pinches, and soon too much basil spoils the dish. Alternatively, having tried one spice, you find one is not enough. You begin to put an ever-increasing diversity of spices in every dish, until the food is no longer palatable.

Another scenario: imagine you love roller coasters. You live near an amusement park equipped with one of the most tortuous and thrilling roller coasters in the country. The first time you go on it, you are scared out of your skin and you *love* it! The next time, it's almost as amazing, the third time it's great, and the fourth time it's okay. By the tenth time it's old hat, and you need to experience new roller coasters to get the same thrill you got the first time you rode the one nearby. You find new ones a little further afield, within a day's drive perhaps. Soon you are planning holidays to far-flung countries for the best roller coaster experiences in the world. Oh my goodness! The thrill of it! The same escalating process can happen with almost anything: car racing, getting tattoos, fitness, sexual partners, base jumping, collecting stamps, making money–the list is almost endless.

So what does this have to do with ADHD and focus? ADHDers have less access to dopamine because of the way their brains process it; when dopamine is released in the ADHD brain, the individual is more affected by it, and finds herself needing ever-more exciting experiences to give her the same rush, making any new or exciting possibility irresistible.

BRANDON BREAKS A HABIT

Brandon came to me because his use (or rather his abuse) of his mobile phone interfered with his ability to do his job effectively. Brandon's boss told him during his yearly evaluation that if he didn't improve his productivity, his job would be at risk. During our first session, Brandon said he sent and received about 200 text messages a day, and could not stop checking his email, which often contained links he felt unable to resist clicking. A quick look at his phone or computer could lead to hours of wasted time.

Brandon and I formulated a strategy to help him use his mobile phone more rationally. First, he agreed to limit the number of times he checked his phone for voice and text messages – down to five from about 100 each day.

Deciding to do this was as far as he got, he told me the next time we met. He was able to defer listening to voice messages, he said, but he just couldn't ignore a text message. The alert sound signaling a text message was simply irresistible. When we explored the issue further, we discovered phone messages were general calls to action: someone wanted him to do something. Text messages, however, usually contained "fun stuff:" humor from friends, or racy suggestions from his girlfriend. It wasn't hard to figure out why he found it tough to leave the text messages unopened!

Our second strategy to keep him from checking the phone was to have him turn it off, and/or leave it in the car. This worked, except he was miserable. He dragged through the day like he was being cheated out of something. He managed to focus more on his work, but his energy and enthusiasm began to wane. Eventually, because he had lost interest, he began daydreaming and once again lost focus.

Being without his phone obviously wasn't the answer for Brandon. But what was?

Brandon isn't the only one to have this type of problem—it may even ring some bells for you. In fact, so many people have similar issues that some interesting research is being done to further explore them. The research indicates dopamine is closely tied to desire, but not just for pleasure. Just as a coffee addict may begin to crave a skinny latte when she walks past a Starbucks, Brandon expected a reward when he heard the text message alert: there was a thrill to be experienced, dopamine to be had! That's why Brandon found the messages irresistible. Conversely, removing the alert sound and the message checking reduced his dopamine "hits" thereby making him feel less energetic and, eventually, less able to focus.[5]

IRRESISTIBLE REWARDS WORK WONDERS

How did Brandon and I use this information to his advantage? And how can it help you?

The release of dopamine in the brain is a powerful motivator. Think of the lengths an addict will go to get his fix. Given that cravings occur in the primitive part of the brain that doesn't respond to logic and reason, denial is often futile, as the primitive part of the brain doesn't listen well. The trick is

---

[5] Kent C. Berridge and Terry E. Robinson, *What is the role of dopamine in reward: hedonic impact, reward learning, or incentive salience?*: Brain Research Reviews, 28, 1998. 309–369.

to use the motivational aspect of dopamine release to achieve a desired behavior. This can be done by using the stimulus/response cycle itself (in this case, text message alert sound leads one to check the message), to create a positive rather than negative result. In Brandon's situation, this meant using the text messages as a reward for focusing on the work he was meant to do, rather than as a distraction from it.

When Brandon heard the text message alert sound, he would finish the page of the report he was working on, or initiate one of the business calls he had to make, or do any other activity that he had difficulty motivating himself to do, before he would allow himself to check the incoming message. Brandon was reluctant to try this at first. He worried it would be torture beyond what he could endure, but he was desperate to keep his job, so he gave it a go. He was surprised to find when he started using this strategy that he enjoyed the anticipation of reading messages more than actually reading them. Upon reflection, this makes sense. Because there is often so little time between stimulus and response in our fast-paced world, we fail to realize the "highs" we get from doing things come from *anticipating* them rather than actually *doing* them.

Once he got in this new groove, Brandon took another step. When working on a boring task, such as reviewing a report, he would think of funny or racy texts to send to his friends and girlfriend, and then make himself complete a certain amount of work before sending them. He found when he rewarded himself for doing small parts of large projects, he was able to more easily complete the entire piece of work. Texting throughout the day, rather than completely denying himself the use of the phone, actually made him more efficient.

MONICA MANAGES HER MAIL

Like Brandon, Monica loved to check emails from her friends, as well as read newsletters and updates to which she was subscribed. She even enjoyed checking her business emails. But she was unable to use them as a focus-inducing reward because they all came into one email inbox, and the business-related emails often included action items needing her attention. She'd think she could answer this or that email quickly, but before she knew it, an hour had passed and she had lost focus on whatever non-email related work she had been trying to complete. The solution for her was to create two email accounts, one for her friends, newsletters, subscriptions etc., and another for business-related matters. Now she could maintain focus (by scheduling when she would check business emails) and motivation (by looking forward to answering emails in the "fun" account at other times). She also reduced the time she spent on email overall.

The reward system is one of the most powerful motivators we have to elicit desired behavior. Using it as a tool to achieve your goals is easier (not to mention much less stressful!) than the arduous battle of trying to change your brain's wiring.

The "carrot on a stick" idiom captures the concept nicely. The story behind the idiom involves a clever cart driver who dangles a carrot on a long stick just out of reach of the donkey harnessed to his cart. As the donkey strains to get at the carrot, it pulls the cart, the driver and the carrot forward. Of course the carrot always remains just beyond reach, and the donkey keeps pulling the cart in an effort to get to it. The moral of the story: it's more sensible to use the fact that donkeys like carrots than it is to try to change the stubborn nature of the donkey. Likewise, it makes more sense to optimize the way our brain is wired than it is to change it.

You too can use these techniques to change your own behavior. Consider which "rewards" might help you through activities you find less enjoyable. Is there a motivator you can incorporate throughout your day? Research tells us that emails, texts, phone calls, and checking the news are at the top of the list of things that distract people from doing what they "*should*" be doing. Nevertheless, reading and writing text messages provided Brandon with the greatest incentive to stay focused. What are your dopamine release motivators? What is irresistible to *you*?

KEY PUZZLE PIECES SUMMARY

1. Multitasking exacerbates the inability to focus–whether one has ADHD or not.

2. The brain is wired to make us both want to repeat things that feel good, and to try new things. It's a paradox!

3. ADHD brains process neurochemicals differently than non-ADHD brains.

4. The release of dopamine in the brain lies behind addictive and pleasure-seeking behaviors.

5. The reward system is one of the most powerful motivators.

Useful Exercises

Use Technology as a Motivator

What is irresistible to *you*? What do you look forward to and enjoy immensely? We've focused on technology, but I encourage you, so long as it doesn't lead to obesity, lung cancer, or rehab, to feel free to choose anything else that can be done throughout the day to keep you motivated. If you don't know where to start, try the examples described here. Turn your phone off or set it so you won't hear whether or not you are receiving texts, voicemails, e-mails, or alerts from your social networking applications. Also, make it so you can't see incoming email messages on your computer. Alternatively, you can make a commitment to yourself to do a certain amount of a necessary task before checking your phone, computer, or networking site. Be sure to have a limit if you're using the social networking site as a reward, such as only checking messages or reading only one page of updates, so that you don't end up distracted off of your original task.

Take Action

Choose something that currently gets you distracted to use as a motivator, such as one of the examples above. Write how you will use this to motivate you, such as checking only after a certain task is completed. Try several actions, to see which is best, or use them together for added benefit:

1. _____

2. _____

3. _____

Notice if this had any positive effects and write them here. The act of writing them acknowledges them on a deeper level, which can assist in motivating you to continue the practice:

1. _____

2. _____

3. _____

Mark here when you have completed 30 days of arranging a motivator around one task each day.

_____Thirty Days Completed

Congratulations!

UNPLUG

Part of effective time management is knowing when to do an activity. It's important to determine when your brain is most effective for particular tasks. During the time that you are best able to do intellectual tasks, unplug the phone or computer, and block out other distractions.

    Rather than allowing yourself to be distracted randomly throughout the day, save checking emails for particular times and making calls for another. After any initial fears of missing something important wear off, many people feel a greater sense of control over their lives, knowing that they can only be bothered at particular times. This should also help to increase your sense of focus and complete tasks more readily.

Take Action

List activities that you need to complete each day. Make a second list of distractions and how you will control them (i.e., emails—check only before work, during lunch, and once in the evening).

Activities to complete

1._____

2._____

3._____

4._____

5._____

6._____

Distractions and how to control

1._____

2._____

3._____

Mark when you have completed 30 days in a row of controlling one distraction.

_____Thirty Days Completed

Bravo—you did it!

CHAPTER 2

Lack of Follow-Through

LACK OF FOLLOW-THROUGH FOLLOWS ADHD CHILDREN INTO ADULTHOOD

As we have learned, ADHDers generally do not follow instructions nor complete tasks. For them, seeing things through to the end is the exception rather than the rule. They also tend to avoid tasks they sense require more mental effort. In short, they struggle to finish the things they start.

The same is true of ADHD adults, but the symptoms are less frequently apparent, partly because adults have more freedom to choose what they wish to do. It's easier for them to avoid what they don't like or don't want to do. No one will "ground" them for not cleaning their rooms for example–they may leave them looking like a cyclone hit forever without having to face any negative consequences.

Based on experience, adults also have a better idea of which tasks they will find more challenging to complete. By taking on fewer of them, they hide their issues with follow-through. However, even "grown-ups" can't choose to *always* avoid *everything* they might not want to do, so their inability to "get the job done" manifests eventually.

Like ADHD children, ADHD adults often do not complete tasks because something else grabs their attention or the details involved in finishing the task overwhelm them. But ADHD adults are more prone to suffer the ill effects of poor organization and time management, having missed out on learning how to organize and schedule skills as children. They often fail assemble all the materials required, for example, or give themselves sufficient time to complete tasks. Thus, while the inability to follow through is a discrete symptom, it frequently results from, and is compounded by, other issues such as being disorganized and inefficiently managing time.

You know as well as I that having ADHD is not a prerequisite for being disorganized. Likewise, lack of follow-through in both ADHDers and non-ADHDers can be caused by a multitude of factors. Some scientists believe the avalanche of fragmented information to which we are exposed adversely impacts our capacity for concentration. Just take a moment to reflect on the number of chunks of "stuff" that bombard your brain when you watch a five-minute music video, the evening news, or spend an afternoon in a shopping mall: millions and millions of sights, sounds, and smells to digest every day! No wonder people (including those who don't have ADHD) are overwhelmed.

One especially worrying aspect of information overload is its potential impact on children's brains during critical stages of development. When children start reading, for example, their brains build pathways that will be used to analyze and comprehend information for the rest of their lives. Some experts are concerned that today's children, who get information in quick, flashy, pre-digested formats, will be less able to analyze complex data and make decisions as adults. Will today's children be able to comprehend information delivered in deeper, more complex forms when they grow up? Will it have to be pre-processed into smaller bites because their brains' analytical pathways were not properly developed in childhood?

Follow-through is about sticking with something when it isn't easy. As we become accustomed to being fed information that doesn't require "chewing" by the brain before it's digested, we may eventually forget how to chew. We may become less adept at figuring things out on our own and more likely to give up on difficult mental tasks. Not a happy prospect in a world where problems of ever-increasing complexity demand that we come up with ever-more-complicated solutions.[6]

That's the "theory." But how do follow-through issues manifest in reality? Joan and Robert are good examples of how a weak follow-through isn't only problematic in tennis and golf. . .

WHY CAN'T I GET IT TOGETHER?

Joan arrived in my office with multiple ADHD-related issues. Chief among them was her inability to finish anything. Her life was like one big ball of yarn from which thousands of loose ends dangled, as if someone had randomly snipped it with scissors. She was easily frustrated and often felt overwhelmed. It seemed that everything was much more difficult for her

---

[6] Malcolm Ritter, *Scientists concerned about effect of technology on brain*, Associated Press, December 3, 2008.

than for others, and the problem caused her to miss out on life experiences she knew she would enjoy if only she could stay in control. Joan avoided travel, for example, because she found it too much effort to pack, arrange transportation to the airport, get there at a particular time, find the right gate, etc. – and then there were all the arrangements to take care of things in her absence!

These tasks aren't a pleasant part of travel for anyone, but for Joan, they were insurmountable. She could not deal with the effort required to concentrate and remember everything, nor with the anxiety of knowing she was likely forgetting something. All of this simply made travel too exhausting to even attempt. She didn't understand why tasks such as these wore her out, yet were seemingly a breeze for everyone else. She often felt inadequate, incompetent, and incapable–not to mention infuriated! "What's wrong with me?" she asked herself in despair.

As we worked together, I carefully reframed Joan's situation for her. We discussed the fact that it wasn't so much that she couldn't manage her life, but rather that her brain functioned differently from others. Modern life is fast, furious and full of information. This can be both good and bad for an ADHDer. On the one hand, when millions of bits of information come at you in swift succession, it can be handy to have a brain that grasps concepts quickly and shifts easily between tasks, as the ADHD brain is well equipped to do. Unfortunately, a plethora of details usually accompanies large volumes of information, and because of the way they process details, ADHDers become overwhelmed by relatively small tasks that others can accomplish with scarcely a second thought.

Why? Because of the way the ADHD brain works. (Remember the bit about the brain in Chapter 1, where we talked about lack of focus? Here we go again. . .)

There is an area at the front of the brain called the *prefrontal cortex*. Among other things, the prefrontal cortex takes in information from the environment and decides what to do with it. Scans that measure brain activity have found the prefrontal cortex works differently in the brains of people with ADHD.

When a "normal" person is given a task to complete and her brain is scanned as she does it, the prefrontal cortex lights up, showing that it is actively processing the information necessary to complete the task. The rest of the brain stays more or less inactive. When such a test is done with a person who has ADHD, the prefrontal cortex does not light up in the same way, indicating it's inactive. However, several other regions of the brain *do* light up, indicating that the ADHDer uses areas of the brain other than the prefrontal cortex to complete the task. In other words, the brain compensates for what the prefrontal cortex in the ADHDer is unable to do. While the person may complete the task, he or she may feel overwhelmed, because the part of the brain doing the work isn't designed to do so.

JOAN'S SECRET STRUGGLES

Joan was not aware of the way her brain compensated for itself; neither were those around her. They could see Joan eventually completed tasks such as paying her bills and doing her grocery shopping, and they didn't understand why she felt overwhelmed by them. Neither Joan nor others could see inside her head, and know the way her brain functions caused her to feel out of her depth (just as others with ADHD do).

So why is it a problem to use areas of the brain other than the prefrontal cortex to complete tasks? A "non-mental" analogy may help to illustrate. Let's say I spill a bag of popcorn on the floor in your living room, and you (an able-bodied person with all appendages intact) have to clean it up. It wouldn't be a big deal, right? But what if you had to pick up each piece of popcorn individually using your feet instead of your hands? You would be able to do it, but it would be difficult and time consuming, because feet are designed to help us walk and balance, not grasp and carry.

Now, imagine every time you enter the living room, you find an increasing number of bags of popcorn emptied on the floor. The first time, one bag. The second time, two. The third time, three. How hard would it be to deal with the mess the tenth time you entered the living room? Even a person who could use his hands to pick up the popcorn might begin to feel frustrated, angry, and discouraged, but likely not to the same degree as she who was forced to pick it up with her feet. Eventually, she might stop going into the living room entirely, because the very thought of all that popcorn would be distressing.

That's how the hassles of daily life felt to Joan. She finished the tasks that required integrating details and making decisions, but each one filled her with dread, and she felt like she was drowning as she did them. Not surprisingly, like a lot of people with ADHD, Joan delayed or did not do those types of tasks. She simply gave up.

For Joan, the analogy of not having the use of her hands to pick up spilled popcorn makes sense, as she sometimes feels "disabled." I prefer the term "differently abled." She may not have the same level of functioning within the prefrontal cortex as a non-ADHDer, but this has forced her to develop other areas of her brain more highly.

Details may be crushing, but she is more able to see the big picture than her work colleagues, and she can generate ideas and solutions to problems long after others' creative juices have run dry. Having been unable to work within the confines of the "normal" box, she is much more adept at thinking "outside of the box," a great gift in a world that constantly demands innovative solutions to challenging problems.

Being differently abled takes many forms. I have another client, Nick, who is a writer. Nick's fingers can scarcely keep up with the volume of ideas he conceives, formulates and records on his computer. When he sits down to write an article, he types at about 50 words per minute. This is the speed at which he generates the idea *and* gets it "down on paper." It's astonishingly fast, even for a top-notch writer. Most of us type at a snail's pace compared to Nick: about 19 words per minute, less than half Nick's breakneck speed is the average pace.[7]

HOW TO GROUP IT TO GET TO IT

Noticing and honoring her special abilities made Joan feel better about herself, but it didn't help her do the many tasks over which she remained overwhelmed. Having identified that detail-heavy tasks exhausted her, Joan and I set out to: 1) reduce the number of these tasks, and 2) decrease the amount of thought each task required.

Luckily, Joan's husband was less bothered by detail than she was. Joan had been loath to ask for his help because she felt she should be able to manage on her own, and she felt stupid having to pass off things that required thought. To maintain her self-esteem, we worked on keeping her challenges in perspective while celebrating her talents. In the end, she felt grateful to her husband for taking on tasks that depleted her energy, and she found other ways to shoulder her share of household management duties.

Nevertheless, Joan still had to complete unavoidable and tiring tasks she was unable to "delegate" to her husband. She put these "hassles" in a separate section on her to-do list, and scheduled them carefully so she didn't have to do too many together. It took some experimentation before she figured out which were particularly difficult and how many she could handle daily. To

---

[7] Karat, C.M., C. Halverson, D. Horn, and J. Karat, 1999, *Patterns of entry and correction in large vocabulary continuous speech recognition systems*, CHI 99 Conference Proceedings, 568–575.

make them more palatable, she sandwiched onerous activities between more invigorating ones—jogging before a task, then doing something relaxing afterwards, for example. By honoring what was difficult for her, she made it much more manageable.

Joan also found that grouping like tasks together made doing them easier. For example, she saved bills in a box as they came in, and paid with them all on Mondays. This system reduced her anxiety because she only had to deal with bills once a week, she wasn't distracted each time one arrived (because she just put it in the box), and she didn't have to worry about any slipping through the cracks. Finally, she became more efficient by keeping everything she needed to pay the bills in one drawer so she didn't have to search for it each time.

Joan's follow-through issues manifested mainly at home. Others, like Robert, experience them primarily at work. Luckily, Robert had a secretary that thrived on feeling needed. When he shared with her that he found some things particularly challenging—tracking down the relevant forms for a particular project and getting them to the right place at the right time, for example—his secretary was happy to help. Once she knew about his ADHD-related issues, she began to find other areas where she could support him. Meanwhile, Robert could do more of the things at which he excelled with the time and energy freed up by his secretary's assistance. Like Joan, he found ways to better manage financial matters: he automated and delegated bill payment through his employer and his bank. As a result of these changes, he felt more in control and competent, instead of lazy and deficient for needing help.

If you experience problems with follow-through, remember there are strategies you (ADHDer or not) can use to get things done. Many of them relate to organizational skills, which we'll discuss in the following chapter.

KEY PUZZLE PIECES SUMMARY

1. Put your talents, abilities and 'shortcomings' in perspective to feel better about yourself.

2. Remember: the inability of ADHDers to follow through is based in brain functioning, not lack of capacity or laziness!

3. Delegate tasks to stop feeling overwhelmed.

4. Reduce the number of tasks and decrease the amount of thought involved in each one.

5. Schedule and group tasks together to better manage them.

Useful Exercises

CREATE "TO DO" LISTS AND CALENDARS (AND DELEGATE WHEN POSSIBLE!)

List making is an essential component of organization. Lists are particularly helpful for decreasing forgetfulness and increasing the likelihood of follow-through. When it is difficult to keep track of details, lists take the thinking out of remembering. By making a to-do list each day, you can see how much needs to be done and allot adequate time to do it.

One way of enhancing a to-do list even further is by dividing up items into what *must* be done and what it would be *nice to do*, or what needs to be done at work versus what needs to be done at home, or even what is enjoyable versus what is draining. By having lists, you never need to worry that you will forget to do something.

Lists can also help you get organized. For example, making a list of work projects will make sure that anything that is needed will get done. A grocery list ensures needed items can be written down, so they will be remembered on shopping day. You can also start lists for holidays or travel items–write things down as they occur to you so you are less stressed trying to remember things at the last minute.

Create your lists in a way that ensures you will look at them. A note-pad on the fridge, a notebook you carry with you, the notes function available on most phones or computers, all work well as long as they are with you when you think of the things you must remember. You may choose to use a combination of strategies for different purposes (e.g. a grocery list on the fridge, an overall to do list on your phone).

If, when you review your lists, you find the number of tasks daunting, it's time to delegate. Ask yourself if there are tasks that could be done as well if not better by someone else. Could the housework be done by a cleaning service? Might your partner pick up the dry cleaning on the way home from work every second Tuesday? Could a team member at work do part of the research needed for an ongoing project? If yes, get those tasks off your lists and onto theirs! Equally, you may also find items on your list that others have delegated to you. Make sure you don't accept tasks if you don't have time to do them: in other words, learn to say no. The objective of delegation is to end up with the tasks that are most suited to our abilities. If you try to do it all, you'll be less effective.

(Continued)

Keep a calendar too. Record in advance what you must remember so you to have all the necessary information when and where you need it on the day. For example, on the date of an event put the event address and location, the venue phone number, what you need to bring, the dress code, etc., to avoid the stress of having to recall it all on the day.

Take Action

Make at least one list each day (e.g. a to-do list, a grocery list), or be more detailed in the calendar that you keep; update your list daily. The more that you practice using a list, the more you will discover ways to make lists work for you. Consistency is the key to success.

Write one area where you will keep a daily list:

1. _____

2. _____

3. _____

Decide the best place to keep your list (e.g. on paper, electronically):

1. _____

2. _____

3. _____

After you've completed 30 days, mark it here. Then, think of other lists that would be helpful and list them.

_____ Thirty Days Completed

Yes! You are a superstar.

Additional lists that would be helpful

1. _____

2. _____

3. _____

CHAPTER 3

Disorganization

OH! TO BE ORGANIZED AT LAST

One of the better-known symptoms of ADHD is disorganization. Most children, whether they have ADHD or not, need help getting organized. However, those with ADHD need *a lot* more help, and, because they don't learn these skills as children, and no one is there to manage for them in adulthood, adult ADHDers are even worse organizers and time managers than many kids. This was surely the case in my life.

When I was a child, and well into adolescence, my mother organized and scheduled my entire life, so much so that I didn't have a clue where to start when I reached adulthood–I was at a complete loss! I couldn't organize my way out of a paper bag as the saying goes. I was constantly late for appointments, meetings and get-togethers (if I remembered them at all). Like most adult ADHDers, my lack of organizational skills significantly impacted my life. I had a hard time keeping my belongings together, I constantly lost things, and important stuff regularly fell through the cracks. It was frustrating.

These days, ADHD sufferers aren't alone in feeling overwhelmed by life! It's a sign of our times that armies of consultants get paid vast amounts of money to "organize" us. They specialize in everything from clearing out cluttered closets to re-shaping our chaotic lives in a way that enables us to actually accomplish something instead of running around like proverbial "chickens with our heads cut off." Getting people organized has become big business because being disorganized is such a common problem. I believe "disorganization-itis" is a symptom of modern-day overwhelm with all the information, activity, and "stuff" available to us.

Research shows the sheer volume of content we expect our brains to process is more than they are designed to handle, particularly when it is transmitted through impersonal channels. Long ago, we got information by word of mouth (yes, there was a time when we had no Internet, TV, or radio!).

Then, communication included a personal connection that helped us process content, contextualize messages and see the impact we had on those with whom we interacted. Much of that richness has been lost in the Internet age.

To manage data in this chaotic environment, our brains default to their primitive regions, because the higher-ordered areas, which are actually designed to handle this *type* of content, are not equipped to process large volumes of it delivered at high speed. So massive amounts of information continuously bypass the higher-ordered areas and go straight to the primitive regions. The outward signs of this phenomenon are subtle; by all appearances we may seem to function quite well. However, the primary responsibility of the primitive area of the brain is survival–it activates the fight, flight, or freeze response when we feel threatened. Continual activation of this part of the brain is unhealthy; it results in chronic underlying stress, so familiar to many of us that we have forgotten what it's like to be relaxed. The ongoing activation of the more primitive parts of the brain leads us to feel deluged and worn out.[8] That's why many non-ADHDers experience ADHD-like symptoms.

In the pages that follow, we'll take a closer look at disorganization and the strategies both ADHDers and non-ADHDers might use to address it.

STUFF, STUFF AND **MORE** STUFF

Being disorganized takes many forms, most of which have to do with "stuff." We can't find stuff, we lose stuff, we forget stuff, we're late for stuff, and we miss stuff entirely! All of this wouldn't be an issue except most of us (with ADHD or without), need to have stuff or do stuff (at least some stuff), to live properly. We need access to the right stuff at the right times, and we need to get stuff done efficiently to live well and prosper. And that's where the problem lies. . .

In previous chapters, we saw how the nature of the ADHD brain creates challenges for ADHDers (of any age) with respect to focus and follow through. The same physiological differences make it hard for them to get and stay organized as adults. Additionally, most ADHDers don't learn organizational skills as children because their lives are often completely orchestrated for them (as mine was by my mother), as they grow up. I know from experience how debilitating disorganization can be.

---

[8] Edward Hallowell, *Harvard Business Review*, January 2005.

As a med student, my typical morning routine involved spending half of my time looking for my purse, keys, and the match to the one sock I wore, and the other half trying to re-find them once I located them. When I finally walked out the door, I should have had everything. But no, several trips back into the house were always required. I would start to apply my makeup in the car, only to realize I'd left behind my mascara and lipstick. I would begin to eat my breakfast, only to realize I didn't have a spoon for the yoghurt. I know you might find it hard to imagine someone would eat and "put her face on" while driving, but it's true, I did it. I even put my hair in curlers and rolled down the windows to "blow dry" it in the wind! After I got to a certain point on my drive, I wouldn't turn back–even if I realized I was wearing mismatched shoes. On one occasion I forgot my shoes completely, and had to buy flip-flops at the pharmacy next to the hospital – I got some strange looks that day I can tell you.

Everybody forgets things. You don't have to have ADHD to be absent-minded. But non-ADHDers are generally able to think systematically and remember what they have temporarily forgotten. Such mental gymnastics either require a type of brain function that isn't available to ADHDers, or leads them to feel swamped if they must do it too often. ADHD sufferers need different strategies to manage forgetfulness–strategies from which non-ADHDers may also benefit.

THINK LESS, NOT MORE

To one extent or another, the most effective ways for the ADHD brain to manage the issue of forgetfulness involve decreasing the amount of thinking the brain has to do.

Like Joan, whom we met in Chapter 2, Trevor loved to travel but hated to pack. He enjoyed the excitement of traveling, but the packing was so defeating that he began to dread taking trips. No matter how hard he tried, he always forgot something. This wasn't such a big deal on a trip home to see the family, where most of what he needed was either provided or could be easily purchased. The problem arose when he went snowboarding (an activity he adored). After purchasing untold numbers of expensive ski gloves, he decided something must be done.

Several people had given Trevor less-than-helpful advice. "You just need to *think* when you pack. Just *think* about what you need," they said. Advice like this can be unbelievably frustrating for ADHDers, who in fact draw on *more* of their brain (i.e. they think harder than others), with *fewer* results. ADHDers actually need to think *less* rather than more.

It's in the Bag!

The strategy Trevor and I devised together made packing easy–because it meant he never had to pack again! He simply gathered all his essential snowboarding stuff and put it in a large bag with his snowboard. Whenever he went snowboarding, he grabbed the bag knowing it contained everything he needed. After each trip, he washed whatever needed cleaning, then *immediately* put it back in the bag. Likewise, if anything had to be refilled (e.g. sunscreen, hand warmers), repaired or replaced, he would do it right away, and then put the item back in the bag where it belonged. He also had a master list (in the bag of course), which he used to double-check everything a few days before he left. (See more about list making at the end of the previous chapter, and in the Useful Exercises section at the back of the book.)

The snowboard strategy worked so well Trevor extended it to other kinds of trips. When he traveled, it was generally for less than a week, so he packed for that length of time. He assembled and bagged a week's worth of toiletries, a week's worth of socks and underwear, and a week's worth of medications. Whenever he went away, these individual bags could be thrown into a suitcase and the items replaced when he came home. Using this system, he only had to think once. As long as he replaced the items he used, he knew he had everything he needed and could enjoy the process of planning a trip, rather than feel anxious about it.

Sarah, a single mother, had little time to travel. She was too busy caring for family of three children while working two jobs on a rotating schedule. She had a hard time remembering which ID badges and materials to bring to her jobs, and found it almost impossible to keep track of what her kids needed for school and extracurricular activities. Her life was a chaotic nightmare.

Like Trevor, Sarah needed to take the thinking out of remembering. She too employed a "bagging" solution. She used two separate handbags (one for each job), and a small zippered pouch, which contained her wallet and items she always needed. As she left the house, she would grab the handbag for the job to which she headed, and throw the zippered pouch into it. Finally! She no longer had to worry about forgetting something she needed for work, because she no longer forgot anything.

Next, we attacked the multiple activities associated with her three school-aged children. An over-sized, color-coded calendar that allowed her to more easily track who was doing what, where and when proved invaluable. Using the calendar as a guide, she prepared the kids' respective backpacks (also color-coded) with whatever clothing, equipment, etc. was required the next day. The big calendar was posted in the kitchen where everyone could easily see and refer to it.

SHOP TIL YOU DROP—NOT!

Chloe's disorganization manifested differently. Chloe is a successful consultant and "fashionista" who spends endless hours in shopping malls searching for bargains and decking herself out in the latest looks. But when she first came to me, Chloe had a major shopping problem that had nothing to do with clothes. She was a master at sniffing out the latest fashions at the best price, but when it came to buying food, she was an unmitigated disaster. Chloe had lost count of the number of times she had gone to the grocery store to get one item and had come back with everything but the item that had prompted the trip. Once in the grocery store, she just couldn't remember what she needed.

In this situation, most non-ADHDers would stop, think and eventually retrieve the forgotten item from the recesses of their memory banks. Chloe's brain, however, didn't recognize there was something to remember. She didn't have the feeling she was missing anything, so there was no impetus for her to try to recall what it might be. Her mind was too preoccupied with the multitude of things vying for her attention in the grocery store aisles to focus on what was required to stock her cupboards. Chloe needed help, and fast!

The solution was simple and straightforward: Chloe needed a shopping list. (List making is essential for someone with ADHD.) Chloe put hers on the refrigerator. Whenever she thought of something she had to purchase, or she ran out of a particular item, she put it on the list. She needed to remember it only long enough to write it down, and then she could happily go on her way, thinking of other things. She also bought a notebook, which she carried all the time, and began keeping a to-do list in it. She found she actually enjoyed the sense of accomplishment she felt when she crossed things off the list.

Using a to-do list also decreased her stress level at work. She had been in the habit of letting other people's interruptions distract her. When colleagues popped into her office with a request, she would interrupt her current task and begin thinking about the new request. Now, instead of immediately switching her focus to the new request, she put it on the to-do list she kept on her desk, and continued what she was doing. She knew she wouldn't forget the new request because it was there on the list. She could figure out the details later, when she had completed her existing task and was ready to move on to something new.

WHAT'S THE BIG "TO DO" ALL ABOUT?

Mohammed, a journalist, was in the same boat as Trevor, Sarah and Chloe. He constantly forgot what he was supposed to do or buy. He would be thrilled with himself when he churned out a great article, then horrified when he realized he'd forgotten to conduct a scheduled call because he got so caught up in his writing. Shopping was equally disastrous. He ran to the store every other day because he never got everything he needed at once. Luckily, he was single with no children, so no one depended on him for food–they would have starved! He kept trying to think harder and remember more, and felt worse when he still forgot everything. As he put it, he was tired of feeling like "an incompetent idiot."

Mohammed tried making lists in the same way Chloe had, but he was in and out of the house so much he never seemed close to his grocery or to-do list when he thought of things he should add to them. He also couldn't seem to remember to take the lists with him when he left the house. But he *always* remembered his mobile phone. Bingo! Rather than keeping paper lists or a notebook, he began using the notes function on his phone.

He kept three main lists: things to buy, things to do for work, and things to do outside of work. Whenever something occurred to him, he keyed it into the relevant list, and then stopped thinking about it. He checked his "to-do" lists first thing each morning, and his "to buy" list when he was at the store. With all his tasks on a neat list, Mohammed was better able to determine when to do each one. Ironically, once he didn't have to think so much, he became more relaxed and was in a better state to remember many of the things he formerly forgot.

UNFINISHED BUSINESS

In addition to list making, better planning also alleviates some of the organizational issues associated with ADHD. Living in "the now" isn't all it's cracked up to be, especially for ADHDers: they tend to live in the moment in a way that is detrimental to getting things done. The latest shiny object flashing in front of them inevitably grabs their attention and draws it away from the last shiny object that captured it. No surprise here! ADHDers are easily distracted and highly likely to avoid anything that requires sustained mental effort.

That's why ADHD adults tend to do simple tasks first and put off those on which they must concentrate heavily. When they finally get to the latter (towards the end of the day), the more "difficult" tasks seem impossible to tackle–hence the huge amount of unfinished business in the lives of ADHD adults. "Wait a minute," you may say, "this happens to lots of people! It's not unique to people with ADHD." You're right; many people who don't have AHDD also find it hard to get things done. What makes the problem different for ADHDers is its root. Once again, to find the root cause, we turn to the brain.

NEUROCHEMICALS AND SLEEP ISSUES

As we saw in earlier chapters, one of the main differences between the ADHD brain and the "normal" brain is the former's inability to effectively use dopamine. Dopamine is the neurochemical that helps us stay energetic, attentive, and focused. It is thought that ADHDers rely more heavily on other neurochemicals such as acetylcholine to concentrate, likely due to due to the reduced capacity of their brains to use dopamine. Acetylcholine is mostly used in the higher-ordered, intellectual part of the brain; it's the neurochemical we all (ADHDer and non-ADHDer alike), use in processes associated with concentration and memory.

Heavier use of acetylcholine may be the reason behind some of the more positive aspects of the "typical" ADHD personality (i.e. a tendency to be highly creative, innovative, social, sensory, and open to new ideas). It may also be why ADHDers enjoy generating ideas and talking about them, thus often disrupting classrooms (as children), and formal meetings and gatherings (as adults).

To make the most of their unique neurochemical situation, ADHDers must make the most of acetylcholine, the levels of which are sensitive to sleep: ensuring one gets adequate rest can increase acetylcholine levels in the brain. Unfortunately, ADHDers are often somewhat sleep deprived, as they can have trouble calming down sufficiently to fall (and stay) asleep.

Sleep issues sometimes lead people (of *all* kinds), to turn to sleeping pills, frequently with counterproductive results. Sleeping pills, particularly over-the-counter ones such as Tylenol PM, decrease the release of acetylcholine in the brain. Even non-ADHDers may find it more difficult to concentrate the day after using this type of medication, although their dopamine may bridge the gap and help them get through the day. For ADHDers, it's a different story–the day after taking something such as Tylenol PM will be very difficult indeed because their brains are unable to access dopamine in the same way as a normal brain (as we discussed in Chapter 1).

Besides sleep, other ways of increasing acetylcholine levels include eating particular types of foods such as fatty meats, nuts, dairy products, and egg yolks, as well as certain vegetables, such as broccoli, zucchini, cucumber, and lettuce. Likewise, different supplements may be helpful. However, as supplements in general are not as well regulated and tested as pharmaceuticals, I am reluctant to make specific recommendations. (See more in *Understanding Treatment Options* towards the end of the book.)

TIMING *Is* EVERYTHING

What do neurochemicals have to do with planning and time management? Well, one of the key components of time management is building a life schedule that maximizes your strengths and mitigates your weaknesses. In other words: choose to do certain tasks at the times during which your physiology is best suited to complete those kinds of tasks. Early risers do their best work before noon, night owls peak between 9:00 p.m. and 2:00 a.m. (that's certainly not me!).

As a rule, because of the way their brains function, ADHDers should choose to do those tasks that require more concentration in the morning. Why? Because acetylcholine levels are normally highest in the morning, and, as we have just seen, ADHD brains tend to rely on acetylcholine for concentration. Putting off tasks that require sustained mental effort is detrimental for ADHDers because they may not have sufficient acetylcholine for the level of concentration required to complete complex tasks later in the day.

By the time an ADHDer forces herself to do the onerous work she has put off, her neurochemical juice is depleted, and her brain lacks fuel. She doesn't leave the job unfinished due to laziness; she simply doesn't have the neurochemical resources at hand to get it done.

HOCUS POCUS HYPER FOCUS!

Remember Nick the magazine writer I mentioned in Chapter 2? The one whose fingers could barely keep up with his ideas? His work requires a lot of concentration. When he first started writing for a magazine full time, he preferred to work at night, when distractions were few. After several months on the job however, he found it more difficult to get motivated in the evening. He started to put his work off, and began to run into trouble making deadlines. As we explored the issue together, we found that, with time, the novelty and excitement of having a job as a writer had worn off for Nick. In addition, his boss had asked him to write a series of articles on topics he found less interesting.

What happened to Nick is quite common with ADHD. As we have already seen, lack of focus (a hallmark of ADHD) seemingly vanishes when an ADHDer latches on to something that interests him. All of a sudden he seems to gain an almost super-heroic ability to hyper focus on the task at hand. (This is how I managed to get through the basic-science years of medical school. A lot of concentration was required, but I was so excited to learn about the human body and how it works that I happily studied for hours on end.) This apparently paradoxical behavior can be extremely frustrating for those close to ADHDers. They notice the ADHDer focus extraordinarily well on some things, and not at all on others.

The phenomenon can be relatively easily understood by looking again at the role of neurochemicals in the brain. Someone with ADHD can concentrate quite well when the activity elevates his dopamine levels. When Nick was excited by his new job as a writer, the thrill of it gave him a dopamine "rush," which in turn enabled him to focus and write late at night. As the excitement lessened, and the dopamine rush subsided, he began to lack concentration and motivation. No matter how hard he tried, his efforts to recapture the thrill of working at his dream job proved fruitless. Once he looked at the problem as a neurochemical management issue, as we did in consultation, he could see how paying attention to how he scheduled his work could make a difference–and lo and behold it did!

In general, unless they are very excited about the task, ADHDers should arrange their to-do lists so they tackle their most difficult, concentration-intensive tasks in the morning. More pleasurable and stimulating activities–such as checking email and social media sites, or making phone calls–should be done when acetylcholine levels dip (i.e. usually in the late afternoon). While it's tempting to check emails first thing in the morning, it's best not to waste precious time when acetylcholine levels are high. Nick found that waiting to look at his emails actually made him get his difficult tasks done *faster*, as he was eager to get through them and see what his inbox contained (remember the reward system we talked about in Chapter 1?). Likewise, Nick began to schedule phone calls (which he enjoyed) later in the afternoon when intense concentration was more difficult for him.

In this highly complex and information-rich world, non-ADHDers can realize huge benefits and be more productive by applying the same kinds of time-management principles. For example, I recommend switching off phones and similar devices, or putting them on silent, within certain time frames. It's amazing how far off track one phone call can take you. Likewise, it's wise to defer checking and answering emails until a specific, scheduled time. I became infinitely more productive when I limited the number of times I checked my email to late morning, lunchtime, and evening, instead of every five minutes! At first I worried it would somehow cause me to miss out or get behind. I was delighted when the most significant consequence was greater productivity. An added bonus was seeing how many things got figured out while people waited for me to reply. I not only better managed the tasks I had, I reduced the tasks requiring my input or effort because other people dealt with them, or they sorted themselves out while sitting in my pending file.

So far we've looked at three of the seven adult symptoms of ADHD: lack of focus, poor follow-through, and disorganization. Next on the list? Social issues, the area in which we see some of the most significant impacts on the lives of ADHDers.

KEY PUZZLE PIECES SUMMARY

1. Today's brains are called upon to process more information than they were designed to handle.

2. Physiological differences in ADHD brains make it challenging for AD-HDers to get and stay organized.

3. ADHDers need to think less not more to function more effectively.

4. "Bagging" and "listing" can help anyone and everyone be more organized.

5. Be aware of timeframes during which you are more and less effective and schedule tasks accordingly.

Useful Exercises

PUT THINGS IN THEIR PLACE

Organizing your belongings will make life easier and less stressful. Imagine eliminating the frustrating experience of not being able to find your keys. Or, think of how much less stressful packing would be if you knew you always had what you needed.

I like the saying "A place for everything, and everything in its place." Having a particular place for everything and returning it to that place when you are done using it means you never have to wonder where it is. Always keep frequently used items such as keys, in the same easy-to-access (a hook by the door for example). If several things are needed each time you go out, have an organizing center (or even just a shelf) by the door. Items placed there will be easily available when you come and go.

Likewise, keeping all the items required for one activity together in one place ensures they're readily available when you need them. For example, if you enjoy skiing, have a box or bag with all your skiing gear–you won't have to search high and low for all your ski stuff the next time you hit the slopes. Having everything you need to pay bills available in one box can also streamline the process when you sit down to deal with your account. Even keeping items in a particular place in your car or purse means always knowing where they are–so long as you return them, of course!

Take Action

List items that you often search for, along with a place where each item can be kept:

1. _____

2. _____

3. _____

List an activity, frequent trip, or place you go that requires you to remember several items. Then write an idea for a way to house all of the needed items together (a box, bag, particular drawer, etc.):

1. _____

2. _____

3. _____

(Continued)

As organizational ideas are widely available, list others here that you know would be helpful, but haven't committed to trying (yet!):

1. _____

2. _____

3. _____

Now, commit to 30 days of: returning an item to a particular place each day, keeping a designated place for items related to an activity, or another organizational idea. The important thing is to commit to daily use of the technique. List what you will commit to doing, and mark when 30 days in a row have been completed:

1. _____

2. _____

3. _____

_____ Thirty Days Completed

I bet you feel more organized already!

SCHEDULE AND MANAGE YOUR TIME

Choosing the best time to complete tasks is a big factor in whether or not (and how well), things get done. ADHDer or not, there are times during the day when the neurochemical milieu of your brain is more conducive to doing certain tasks rather than others.

There are two key components to time management: knowing what needs to be done, and determining when to do it. Generally, we tend to figure out what needs to be done and how long each item will take, and then we start going about doing those items. If, however, we also think about the best time to do each item, we can complete them more efficiently, using less energy. If you are most able to concentrate in the morning, it may be best to save tasks requiring concentration to the following day, rather than struggling to complete them in the afternoon or evening. If a task is pleasant, it might be best to do that task at a time when your energy is lowest, when you are less able to do other tasks.

Take Action

List tasks you must do during a typical day. For example, returning calls/emails, particular tasks at work, home-related tasks, paying bills, etc.:

1. _____

2. _____

3. _____

4. _____

5. _____

6. _____

7. _____

8. _____

9. _____

10. _____

11. _____

12. _____

(Continued)

Using the list above, group the tasks according to when it is best for you to complete them.

Morning tasks

1. _____

2. _____

3. _____

During-work tasks

1. _____

2. _____

3. _____

Right-after-work tasks

1. _____

2. _____

3. _____

Evening

1. _____

2. _____

3. _____

Arrange your tasks daily for 30 days. It might take several tries before you know when the best time is for a particular task. Not to worry; what is important is developing an awareness of your own ideal schedule and then consistently applying it.

_____ Thirty Days Completed

Well done!

CHAPTER 4

Social Issues

SOCIAL MISFIRES BEGET SOCIAL "MISFITS"

ADHD behavior, which may sometimes seem bizarre, erratic and incomprehensible to non-ADHDers, makes "fitting in" and interacting effectively with others a real challenge for ADHDers. In general, people with ADHD find relationships and the social landscape of which they are a part difficult to navigate.

Relationships are complicated. Add ADHD symptoms, and a lack of social skill development in childhood to the mix, and they become even more so. Appearing not to listen, interrupting others, having difficulty waiting your turn, leaving things unfinished, forgetting and losing stuff, not showing up for appointments, and living in chaos are behaviors frowned upon by the world at large, and impact how well (or more to the point, how *poorly*), ADHDers relate to others.

Problematic communications often push others away from those with ADHD. Non-ADHDers are accustomed to others making eye contact and listening more or less attentively during conversations, and may feel disrespected when ADHDers repeatedly avert their gaze or interrupt. Non-ADHDers may also expect ADHDers to follow through on what they are asked to do. Rather than make allowances for an ADHDer's diversity of "handicaps," a non-ADHDer may decide instead to end a friendship or relationship.

As a result of deficient social skills, ADHDers may damage their deepest family relationships, and be further hurt by not receiving the full benefits of friendships as well as romantic and collegial relationships.

Obviously, adults with ADHD aren't the only ones who lack social skills and have relationship issues. In fact, some researchers believe our increasing use of technology is adversely impacting our collective ability to socialize. Gary Small, a psychiatrist at the University of California, Los Angeles, has done some fascinating research in this area. His findings show the more we use our brains on technology-related activities, the less we interact with "real" people; and the less we interact with real people, the worse we become at meaningful engagement. Much of the nuance of communication is nonverbal, and face-to-face interaction is critical to developing good interpersonal skills. The ability to read facial expressions and body language is a basic human skill and a pre-requisite for healthy communication.

As we become increasingly proficient at multitasking while 'chatting' online or talking on the phone, the harder it may be to *not* multitask when we talk face to face. Most of us are now accustomed to glancing away from our work to check emails, text messages, and phone call alerts, and we do it automatically during face-to-face encounters when it's inappropriate to do so. It's a pity because multitasking during conversation disrupts the emotional connection between the conversants.[9]

Open Mouth, Insert ADHD Foot

Impulsive behavior is another way in which ADHD negatively impacts communication. ADHDers tend to speak spontaneously, without first processing their words through the prefrontal cortex, the higher-order-thinking part of the brain. This sounds to the listener like the ADHDer has given little thought to what he is saying, which in a sense is true.

In a non-ADHD brain, the prefrontal cortex acts like a kind of communication "gatekeeper." It considers the desired action (i.e. making a statement), and integrates it with other knowledge about the situation, such as what the receiver would like to hear, how the statement might potentially impact the receiver, whether the statement is appropriate for the situation, etc. After processing the data, it evaluates the wisdom of speaking the words, *then* decides whether to speak the words or not. This sequence does not occur in the ADHD brain, with predictably unpredictable results!

In conversation, an ADHDer may seem impatient, almost irritated with how long it takes her fellow conversant to form a sentence. She jumps in to answer questions before they are fully formulated; she looks around, checks her phone, and gets distracted by noises or people in the environment. Furthermore, her intermittent responses may seem completely unrelated to the topic at hand. In fact, ADHDers often speak in what appear to non-ADHDers to be unrelated sentences, leaving the latter baffled with respect to the meaning of what has been

---

[9] Malcolm Ritter, "Scientists concerned about effect of technology on brain," the Associated Press, December 3, 2008.

said. As you might imagine, chaotic exchanges of this type are challenging for all concerned, and the resulting disjointed communication is one of the most obvious challenges associated with the social side of life with ADHD. Let's look at some real-life examples of how this manifests in ADHDers.

Neither Willem nor Greg had developed good communication skills in their youth. They frequently interrupted others, blurted out whatever was on their minds, and felt compelled to speak before conversations became too complicated. They were also easily distracted and often responded inappropriately to others. These behaviors, of which neither was aware, had become deeply ingrained.

Had they not had ADHD, Willem and Greg would have learned, over their lifetimes, which styles of communication worked for them, and they would have adjusted the way they spoke accordingly. Unfortunately, that didn't happen due to their ADHD, and, as a result, their poor communication skills wrought havoc in their lives.

Once aware of the importance of good communication (and the communication styles they *didn't* want), they learned more effective ways to interact, and radically changed the way they communicated overall.

WILLEM PAYS THE ADHD PIPER

Willem's former wife Anika quickly tired of the way he communicated–or rather *didn't* communicate from her perspective! It felt to her that Willem was totally disinterested in what she said. She wanted a life partner who *listened* when she spoke so she wouldn't have to turn to friends to enjoy meaningful conversations.

To be fair, it wasn't that Willem didn't value what Anika had to say. On the contrary, he wanted to converse with her–she was his wife after all. But he wasn't aware when his attention shifted, nor why she interpreted it to mean he wasn't listening. Yes, he often interrupted her, but it was because he already knew what she was going to say. He only needed to hear a few words to figure out what would come next, he could easily sing along with a song he'd heard only once, and he could answer questions before they were fully asked. He felt these were unique skills, which improved rather than hindered communication efficiency. It's true that even non-ADHD brains can comprehend what is being said four to five times faster than the rate at which most of us speak.[10] However, the majority of non-ADHDers understand the importance

---

[10] David Swink, Put that iPhone down, I'm talking to you, *Psychology Today*, April 14, 2010.

of allowing others to complete their sentences in conversation. Had Willem understood it too, he would have known Anika wasn't as interested in his responses as she was in feeling needed and heard.

To Willem, however, it made perfect sense to respond to Anika before she finished speaking. He tried to understand her frustration, but couldn't. If someone interrupted him, he didn't even notice; he was usually ready to move on to the next thought anyway. He recognized he became slightly impatient when she spoke, but it was because he wanted to respond, not because he wasn't interested in what she had to say. If he waited until she was done, he might forget what he wanted to say! Also, Willem sometimes felt he was drowning in the detail of Anika's stories. He couldn't determine which bits were important, and he felt anxious trying to listen to everything. When Willem began taking medication, Anika found it easier to converse with him. (He didn't notice any difference at all; he just knew his wife wasn't getting as upset anymore.) They also saw a therapist who pointed out to Willem that communicating is as much about listening as talking. . .

Unfortunately, Anika left Willem in the end, saying his symptoms had become intolerable habits. Willem knew there was some truth to her complaints, and he continued to take partial doses of his "meds," even after Anika left. Sadly, it was too little, too late.

Willem eventually accepted that his inadequate communication skills were largely responsible for the failure of his marriage. People just don't like being interrupted no matter how much they love you!

Presence Makes Perfect (Almost)

After analyzing the communication issues that had led to Willem's marriage breakdown, we came up with a plan for change.

First, he would develop a sense of presence. Many people had complained he seemed distracted when he spoke with them (his wife wasn't the only one). He knew the behavior to which they referred. His eyes were frequently drawn away from whoever he was speaking with to something else in the environment. Willem didn't think this interfered with his ability to listen, but he'd been told countless times others didn't like it. But when Willem tried to listen more, he felt distracted by paying too much attention to listening! He wished he could just be himself without his focus being diverted or others becoming upset.

In order to become more "present," Willem needed to understand what being present in a conversation really meant. "What makes you feel heard

Willem?" I asked. He thought for a while, then answered: "You know, I feel most heard by people who are similar to me. People who just seem to 'get me.'" He noticed, he said, there were particular friends with whom good communication was easy. They grasped what he said with only a few words of explanation.

"How do you know they 'get you?'" I explored further. "If I were watching from the outside, what behaviors would I see that would tell me a friend understood what you were saying?" Willem answered concisely: "When people nod their heads or say something encouraging like 'I know what you mean.'"

Did Willem do this? I pondered. He said he wasn't quite sure. He hadn't monitored his own behavior. I shared my observation that he occasionally nodded or said something like "so that's why" when he was excited about the process in our sessions. This is how I knew he had understood me, and was affected by what I told him. This type of affirmation felt good, and made me want to continue our conversation. I noted too, that if he did it with me, I imagined he did it with others as well.

Willem was relieved he was doing something right, and patted himself on the back for doing it naturally as well. Being eager to change, he vowed to put more such statements and gestures into every conversation; he even decided to make a list of possible gestures to which he could refer. I wondered aloud how present he could be if he consulted a list of gestures like a cheat sheet. It didn't seem a good solution for someone who found the communication process daunting and tiresome. We re-examined his conversations with me, and agreed he didn't need lists of encouraging statements or gestures when we talked–they came naturally because he was interested in what I had to say. Instead of using lists of gestures, I suggested he approach conversations believing the speaker had something worthwhile to say and the exchange would be interesting. Using these strategies, Willem began to be present, instead of distracted, with others.

MIRROR, MIRROR IN YOUR MIND

Presence is so important to awareness and communication that it's worth spending a bit more time discussing it. One can be present in one's own life by noticing and accepting what occurs in each moment. But how can we get out of our own heads and be truly present to the speaker when we're involved in a conversation?

Willem felt most heard by those who "got him." We feel understood by others when they enter our world, that's what "getting" us means. For others to feel that Willem got them, he needed to leave his world and focus on being in theirs, at least during conversations.

According to research, one technique good listeners use to get into others' experience is "mirroring" (i.e. they adopt the facial features and gestures of the people with whom we speak). You have surely done it yourself without being aware of it. Next time you're at a birthday party, take a look around the table when the birthday boy or girl is about to blow out the candles. Often, others will purse their lips as though they were blowing too. Contagious yawning is another example of unconscious mirroring. When someone yawns, it causes a chain reaction of yawning around them. We mirror instinctively during conversations. Have you smiled in kind when someone laughs or grins at you as they tell a joke? Or crossed your arms without thinking when a fellow conversant crosses theirs? You were mirroring!

Why does mirroring make for good communication? For one, it forges a connection between the speaker and the listener: it helps the listener better understand the speaker and makes the speaker feel more "heard." When the body language and gestures of the listener don't match those of the speaker or the speaker's message, a disconnect occurs. For example, smiling, standing straight, and scanning the room while someone tells you a sad story is inappropriate; those kinds of responses may result in you being thought insensitive, unsympathetic and inattentive. If, on the other hand, you slump along with the storyteller's drooping shoulders, it may help you to empathize more fully with how the storyteller feels—heavy and defeated. Likewise, the storyteller is likely to feel you are listening.

Mirroring made sense to Willem, and he used it to improve the quality of his interactions with others. He became more present during conversations by adopting the gestures and mirroring the posture of those with whom he engaged. He took it a step further with people close to him, and mirrored their breathing. This helped him feel what they were feeling, and got him out of his own head at the same time. Rather than deciding to do particular gestures of his own, he simply followed along and "imitated" his co-communicators. He observed and followed, instead of focusing on whether he looked like he was listening or on what the speaker might want him to do.

GREG: FROM CLASS CLOWN TO CLASS BORE?

Greg is a good example of how impulsive communication manifests in real life. Greg returned from a high school reunion feeling low. As an undiagnosed ADHD adolescent, he had been the "class clown," who voiced the first thing that popped into his head. Though he was frequently in trouble with teachers, and struggled to get by academically, he remembered his high school years fondly. He loved being the funny guy, the life of the party. He lived for cracking up the class with witty comments that surprised even him. Yes, he had difficulty concentrating, but he loved what his mind came up with on the spur of the moment. Deep down, he was actually quite shy, and probably wouldn't have spoken up at all if it hadn't been for this impulsivity. He felt clever when he spoke without thinking, and if he consciously slowed himself down, he seemed unable to be the comic who made people laugh.

At the reunion, people greeted Greg with excited looks of anticipation—expecting him to be the funny man they had once known. But Greg, who had been diagnosed with ADHD in adulthood, now took medication to manage his symptoms. He felt unable to deliver witty, funny and spontaneous comments on the spur of the moment as he had done so easily in his youth. His tongue seemed frozen and his brain was in a fog. He had a few drinks to try to get back into his groove, but to no avail. He felt like a cardboard cutout of himself.

Greg had been taking ADHD medication for several years, but now questioned if he really wanted to be medicated down to what felt like a virtual stop. "Do I really want to so average, when I could full of life like I used to be?" he asked himself. Being reminded of the vibrant person he had been as a teen made him wish he wasn't on medication for ADHD as an adult. He began to question what else he might be missing. He wondered, for example, if he could generate more ideas at work, and be more successful if he wasn't so "slowed" by his meds. He gave the issue a lot of thought, and he and I discussed the advantages and disadvantages of ADHD medication: though he had made people laugh with his impulsive quips, his behavior had not supported his academic aspirations; he remembered the funny stuff he said in class, but none of the lessons; he generated what he thought were great responses, but remembered little of what others said; he delighted in what he *put out*, but *missed out* on taking anything in.

Eventually, Greg came to the conclusion that for him, it was a question of balancing the "downside" of taking medication with the benefits he was afforded by doing so.

"EVERY DAY, IN EVERY WAY, I'M GETTING BETTER."

Nevertheless, Greg wasn't terribly enthusiastic about staying on his ADHD meds. He felt he was doing "the right thing" to suppress what he liked best in order to keep from upsetting others and missing out on what they were trying to tell him. No wonder he wasn't excited about treatment. We decided it would be in his best interest to shift away from that perspective, and to reframe taking medication in a more positive light. We chose to use affirmations to help him see his life differently.

An affirmation is a present-tense statement, which describes a desired outcome. For example, a popular one is: "every day, in every way, I'm getting better." By repeating the statement each day (sometimes several times a day), the affirmer experiences the positivity and uplift it contains, and puts herself in a place (an energetic space if you will) to receive the desired benefits. Living life trying to figure out how to suppress his true self in order to be the way others wanted him to be had taken Greg out of the energetic space of being the person *he* wanted to be. He needed to figure out the best of who he could be, and get back into the energetic space of being that person.

To do this, Greg wrote a list of personal characteristics he felt made him special when he was off medication; it included being able to think fast and come up with witty statements and great ideas. He also listed what was good about being on medication to control the symptoms of ADHD—namely: he was calmer and less impatient when talking to people, and he didn't have to keep undoing the damage of making thoughtless statements. Next, he took aspects from each list and combined them to make an affirmation of who he wanted to be. The result was several statements such as this:

"I calmly receive what others say, knowing the right witty statement and great idea will come to me."

This felt right to Greg. Imagining himself to be as described in this affirmation made him feel good, as well as hopeful. He agreed to repeat it several times daily. He also made copies and stuck them in highly visible places so he was frequently reminded of who he was becoming. He knew it would take time for the affirmation to become the truth, if it ever would, but it created a clear goal for him, made him feel more positive and infused him with the belief that change was possible.

As he repeated the affirmation over several weeks, Greg's hopefulness continued to grow. Still, he felt the need for something more. The affirmation made him feel better, but he had trouble translating it into action. In particular, he struggled with calmly receiving what others said. Rather than being calm, he felt increasingly anxious as others spoke. It was simply too much effort to focus on the details of what was being said, *and* monitor his own behavior to ensure it appeared to others he was listening so they wouldn't get upset if he looked like he wasn't! *Plus*, he felt pressured to "think up" a brilliant idea or witty quip, since he couldn't count on spontaneous statements to just flow directly from his brain to his mouth. Phew! He felt totally out of his depth.

Is There an Echo in Here?

Like Willem, Greg needed to become more "present" in conversations, and he also began to physically mirror others to enhance the effectiveness of his communication. But this, he pointed out to me, wouldn't help with the other part of his communication issue—creating a good response. What, Greg asked, could he do? Luckily, another type of mirroring–verbal mirroring–helped Greg improve that aspect well. Verbal mirroring is the best tool to use when it's critical for those with whom one is engaged to know they have been heard.

A practical example of verbal mirroring is the rigorous communication between air traffic controllers and pilots. They can't afford to misunderstand each other because the safety of hundreds of people depends on their ability to communicate clearly and concisely. When air traffic control gives an instruction to a pilot, the pilot repeats the instruction verbatim, *word for word*, to show he has received and understood the message. Synthesizing a response takes too much time, and doesn't assure an exact understanding the way using the same words does. In normal conversation, it would be strange to repeat exactly what our co-communicators say. It's best to pick out one or two key words and *paraphrase rather than parrot* one's response.

Greg practiced verbal mirroring with great success. As others spoke, he listened for key words indicating how they felt. Without sounding like a robot, he used their words in his answers. If a friend mentioned how frustrated he was, Greg formed a simple response around the word "frustrated," something like: "Wow! That must be really frustrating for you." When his boss asked Greg to lead an office improvement project, he repeated back the request. When Greg mirrored others verbally in this way, they knew he was listening to them. His friend understood that Greg empathized with his frustration, and his boss knew Greg clearly understood what was being asked of him.

By focusing on key words to repeat, rather than thinking of what to say, Greg avoided getting caught up in his own head or distracted by things around him. Mirroring also added a step in the process, thereby buying him time to come up with an idea to easily carry on the conversation. He still missed how rapidly his brain had generated responses, but slowing down the process of conversing resulted in reasonably good ideas. He also noticed others seemed pleased they were heard, and the content of his responses were less important to them than he had thought. In addition, his responses no longer seemed random and unrelated to what the others said–conversations flowed and progressed logically instead of jumping all over the place.

Willem and Greg had to practice being present and mirroring (both physically and verbally) when they communicated; it surely didn't come naturally. They quickly realized they didn't need to purposefully use mirroring all the time. They rarely used it with close friends, for example, because they didn't feel the need to. But they appreciated having a skill they could employ when they became anxious about their ability to communicate effectively, regardless of when or where the anxiety surfaced.

The more Willem and Greg used their newly acquired skills, the easier it became to do so. Even the quality of their interactions with difficult co-workers and family members improved. The good news is anyone (including you!) can add mirroring to their communication tool kit and enhance the way they engage others–try it and see for yourself!

KEY PUZZLE PIECES SUMMARY

1. A lack of social skills (not learned in childhood), may negatively impact adult ADHDers' abilities to successfully engage others.
2. Communication is much more than talking; actively listening to others makes them feel heard.
3. Practice physical and verbal mirroring skills to improve your communication.
4. Be more present: it helps you to engage in your life and connect in more meaningful ways with those around you.
5. Choosing to take medication for ADHD often involves compromises.

Useful Exercises

CREATING AFFIRMATIONS

If your way of being with others doesn't seem to work for you and you want to change, it is helpful to affirm the way you desire to be. Often, when people decide something needs to be changed about themselves, they start by focusing on what is "wrong." This is less effective and less motivating than focusing on the positives.

Affirmations are powerful change-makers. Why? Because the brain does not know whether we are *actually* experiencing something or just *thinking* about experiencing it. That's why athletes "practice" a routine in their minds before they actually perform it. Visualizing a great outcome helps increase their chance of achieving it. In the same way, making an affirmation of the way you want to be helps you to experience that way of being in your mind and increases your chances of actually becoming that way.

Not using this powerful ability of our minds to change our lives is akin to taking a long journey by car and only using first gear. We may eventually reach our destination, but the drive will be slow and inefficient. To engage all the gears in your life journey and experience a different way of being, utilize your brain's ability to imagine yourself acting from your desired state of being.

Once you know the way you would like to be, create a statement describing it. One of the most famous affirmation statements is "every day, in every way, I'm getting better." Make sure that the statement is in the present tense and positive—i.e., affirming what you do want, rather than saying what you don't want. Repeat it aloud several times a day, every day, forever!

Take Action

Take a few minutes to do a meditation. Close your eyes and imagine yourself acting from the way you want to be. This may be happier, calmer, or any other way you choose. Make sure you draw in as many senses as possible to get into your desired state. Imagine how things would look, sound, smell, and feel. Write a description of your desired state here:

_____

_____

_____

(Continued)

_____

_____

Create an affirmation statement that captures your desired state. Make sure it is in the present tense and states what you do want, rather than what you don't want (e.g. "I feel confident and comfortable making presentations," NOT "I don't want to feel afraid of public speaking"). Write your statement here:

_____

_____

_____

_____

_____

Commit to stating your affirmation several times per day. It helps to write the statement down on cards and place them in the bathroom, on the refrigerator, and in other places where you will see and read the statement often.

Mark here after you have said your affirmation at least once daily for 30 days.

_____Thirty Days Completed

Congratulations on getting better every day!

COMMUNICATE MORE EFFECTIVELY BY MIRRORING

Good communication skills do not necessarily come naturally for anyone, but can be particularly difficult for those who have had to deal with impulsivity and attention deficit in their formative years. Much has been written on this topic, and many resources are available; here are a few ideas to get you started:

It is important to listen when someone else speaks. Looking at this from the perspective of social skills, it is equally important that the speaker feels listened to. Using mirroring is one way of making speakers feel heard. Mirroring can be done both nonverbally and verbally.

Nonverbal mirroring involves imitating the facial expressions, posture, and mannerisms of the speaker. Try also to match their tone of voice, volume, and speed. The goal is to feel others' experiences. (Hint: don't get so involved in trying to imitate that you let yourself get distracted from what is being said.)

Verbal monitoring is also useful. Listen to the words the speaker uses and incorporate some of them into your answers. Listening to the words uses a different part of the brain than the part that creates a response. Often, while someone speaks, we engage the part of the brain that analyzes and creates a response; this prevents effective listening. By listening for the words to mirror, we hear what is being said before we develop our response. This improves listening, makes others feel heard, and leads to more effective communications with others.

Take Action

Practice mirroring. This may be most effective with a friend or someone else whom you trust to give you good feedback, but you can also practice on strangers, or even using the TV. Write the situations you attempted, along with how effective they seemed, here:

_____

_____

_____

_____

_____

After you've gained comfort with mirroring verbally and nonverbally, commit to doing it at least once daily for 30 days to hardwire it into your brain

(Continued)

and create a natural way of being. Write examples of what you did, and when you've completed 30 days.

_____

_____

_____

_____

_____

_____Thirty Days Completed

Mirror, mirror on the wall, YOU have become the greatest listener of all!

CHAPTER 5

Emotional Reactivity

THE TICKING TIME BOMB OF EMOTIONAL REACTIVITY

Whereas the ADHD symptoms we've covered in the previous chapters (decreased focus, lack of follow-through, disorganization, and social issues) are relatively easily defined, the next area, emotional reactivity, also known as emotional lability, is a bit more nebulous. Still, it's an important, perhaps even *the* most important piece of the ADHD puzzle.

Emotional reactivity, or lability (that's right *lability*, not *liability*, although being emotionally labile can surely be a liability at times), may be the most difficult and damaging of the symptoms experienced by adult ADHDers. It can be hard to understand, not only for the one who suffers it, but also for those in relationship with them. Wisegeek.com gives this layperson's explanation of emotion lability:

> "The symptoms of emotional lability might vary among individuals and in frequency of occurrence. Fits of laughter or crying jags are two examples. Some people do evidence this most with explosive tempers, and there can be instances where people will experience all three emotionally excessive expressions at varied times. When these expressions occur, it's often daunting for the people undergoing them because many people know that their emotional response is in excess to the circumstances. It can even get embarrassing for some individuals or be a condition that makes them withdraw socially."

Emotional reactivity can lead to behavioral issues in children and emotional issues in adults. As we saw in the overview, emotional reactivity manifests in children as temper tantrums or highly energized, sometimes even violent outbursts. In some adults, it can look the same; rather than digesting what is said or happening at a particular moment, emotionally reactive AD-HDers may fly off the handle unexpectedly. Even adults who have learned to suppress these behaviors may still have underlying restlessness, agitation and anxiety.

Adult ADHDers need constant stimulation to function, and may be the life of the party when they're "up." Without stimulation, however, they can feel, and appear, down or depressed. The subtle environmental changes that trigger either "life of the party" or "my life is a disaster" often go unnoticed by others, and the subsequent ADHD-induced mood swings therefore seem totally random. Also, as many other mental health conditions involve extreme moodiness, it may be challenging for health practitioners to diagnose its cause as ADHD, often leading to an incorrect diagnoses of anxiety, depression or bipolar disorder.

Why do ADHDers experience this emotional reactivity? Because, in addition to being restless and stimulation hungry, ADHDers tend also to be highly impatient. The least little bit of frustration can easily set them off, causing them to explode when things don't go their way.

It was this anger and volatility that led Paulo's ex-wife Maria to insist he get help. When frustrated with his computer, he threw it against the wall, as a child might do. Maria never knew when he would break something that he found irritating to use. Though he was never violent towards her, she was still frightened, of his out-of-proportion out-of-control reactions. We'll come back to Paulo later. . .

As with other symptoms such as decreased focus, disorganization and the like, emotional reactivity and the behaviors associated with it may not necessarily be ADHD-related. There are plenty of non-ADHDers who don't handle frustration well and are emotionally volatile. Likewise, there are other mental health conditions that result in these types of behaviors.

Additionally, our use of technology may negatively impact our capacity for control when we feel frustrated. One study involving teenagers demonstrates this well. Researchers had teens play either a violent or non-violent video game for 30 minutes. The brains of those who played the violent game showed more activation in the emotional areas of the brain and less in the higher-ordered areas involved in self-control. It's unknown if playing violent video games might lead to low frustration tolerance in the long term, but it is certainly thought provoking, and worthy of further investigation. By consistently activating the emotional areas without building up those involved with self-control, could we be promoting, in non-ADHDers, the kind of emotional lability and low frustration tolerance seen in those who have ADHD? Only more research will provide the answers.[11]

Now let's take a closer look at how emotional reactivity manifests in real life.

Understanding Jessica's Moods

Jessica had always been considered moody. She felt an almost constant irritability, which was impossible to explain to those around her, partly because she herself could not put her finger on what the problem was. She was upset by something new and different on a daily basis. She overreacted to individual circumstances, but didn't know why this happened or how to stop her behavior. Compounding the problem was the speed at which it occurred; she reacted to things before she even realized what was going on. Her moods worsened as she felt more and more hopeless about ever being "normal." After several well-meaning friends suggested she must be depressed, she was evaluated and treated for depression; but the treatments for depression didn't work. Eventually, after Jessica was correctly diagnosed with ADHD and treated for it, her underlying irritability subsided, as did her over-reactivity.

What Jessica experienced is common in ADHD. However, because irritability and moodiness can also be manifestations of mood disorders (as mentioned above), ADHD is often misdiagnosed as another illness with similar symptoms. The mood issues observed in adult ADHDers are commonly grouped under the term "affective lability," which means their moods are unstable, and quickly shift from "normal" to excited, angry or depressed, either with or without any apparent trigger for the change. In other words, those experiencing the mood swings may or may not be able to identify their cause. It's not unusual for them to experience reactions as being completely spontaneous and unrelated to any external stimuli or event. Furthermore, the intensity of the moods seems excessive or inappropriate compared to events that may have provoked them. A relatively insignificant stressor (misplacing one's eyeglasses, for example) to which a "normal" person would scarcely react, might cause an ADHDer to feel deeply anxious, depressed, or angry. Unfortunately, the intensity of the reaction only exacerbates the problem, requiring

---

[11] Radiological Society of North America, "Violent Video Games Leave Teenagers Emotionally Aroused," *ScienceDaily*, retrieved November 17, 2010, from http://www.sciencedaily.com/releases/2006/11/061128140804

the ADHDer to focus on dealing with the overwhelming emotions, rather than on developing the skills needed to manage the stressors less emotively.

Paulo Is Out of Control

Emotionally labile Paulo, who I mentioned earlier, always felt extremely angry. He was easily irritated, and often exploded in tempestuous outbursts, which, though short-lived, caused significant problems. He was unable to control his overwhelming frustration with anything and everything. He felt so helpless and outraged when something didn't work properly that he had destroyed several pieces of electronic equipment by throwing them against the wall. He wasn't aware of what he was doing while he was doing it. Realization came only when he saw the object of his anger lying in pieces on the floor, at which point he felt ashamed as he dealt with the outcome of his behavior. He felt even worse when someone else, such as his wife Maria, witnessed one of his "tantrums."

Paulo knew he was out of control, but couldn't explain why frustration was so much more difficult for him to handle. An anger management class helped somewhat. He learned to count to 10 before he reacted, which slowed him down, but didn't always stop him. He also learned to verbalize and imagine what he was about to do before he did it. For example, he would say out loud: "I'm going to throw my laptop against the wall," which forced him to imagine his excessive action before he actually did it.

While these strategies were useful, they did not rid him of the underlying feeling that led to him react in the first place. He couldn't relate to the others in his anger management group because he didn't identify himself with feeling angry. Rather, he went from being generally happy, to frustrated then enraged, in an extremely short time. He noticed his over-reactions seemed to occur more frequently when he felt helpless. He wondered if feeling helpless might be related to a lack of life skills, resulting from years of living with ADHD.

I congratulated Paulo on his willingness to explore anger management, and on his successful implementation of the skills he learned. I also told him I felt his reactivity issues were ADHD-related as low frustration tolerance is a hallmark symptom of ADHD. Just as ADHDers easily give up on or avoid challenging tasks, they also often fail to effectively deal with the frustrations of everyday life. Many ADHDers alternate between being immediately able to do something and giving up on the task completely–there's no middle ground. When a non-ADHDer encounters a frustrating situation, he might analyze the problem from several angles and try various solutions to resolve it. An ADHDer, on the other hand, will likely give up if he doesn't see an immediate solution to the problem. If the frustration is unavoidable, such as needing computers to *not do* what computers are renowned for doing (i.e. crashing!), and is combined with the learned helplessness associated with a lack of skills and/or a history of having others figure things out for him, the situation simply overwhelms the ADHDer and causes him to explode–as it did repeatedly with Paulo.

EMOTIONS IN THE BRAIN

Might brain functioning be tied to reactivity? (Having gotten this far in this book, you can probably guess the answer!) When we get upset, the emotional *'fight or flight'* center of the brain called the *amygdala*, is activated. We then either *react* from this primitive area of the brain (i.e. go into fight-flight-or-freeze mode) or *respond* from the higher-ordered, more intellectual area of the brain, called the *prefrontal cortex*. This more developed center of the brain considers options and *then* decides how to proceed. The altered functioning of the ADHD brain makes its more responsive, higher-ordered part less available for use. Without its input, ADHDers instantly react from the amygdala. The ability to utilize the higher-ordered part can be greatly enhanced by medication treatment. Paulo, who took ADHD medication, noticed it improved his concentration and focus, both of which are provinces of the higher-ordered portion of the brain. But he still reacted from the primitive part when he felt frustrated. Why?

The brain is made up of cells known as neurons. When triggered by an experience, neurons release certain neurochemicals, which are sensed by other neurons. This is how they communicate with one another. After repeated experiences, neurons arrange themselves so the message from one is consistently received by a particular other, creating a pathway. The pathway is then followed again when the same experience is perceived. The more any given pathway is utilized, the stronger it becomes and the easier it is to use again.

While this is more efficient, it also results in experiences leading to automatic reactions. For Paulo, and others like him, the pathway for frustrating stimuli is simple: activation of the emotional brain leads to anger and/or explosive outbursts. When emotionally activated, the human brain (no matter whose) tends to react quickly, and uses whichever pathway is easiest. When someone is unaccustomed to engaging the intellectual part of his brain to make conscious choices about how to act, the easiest pathway inevitably leads to primitive unconscious reactions, as with Paulo.

A good analogy is cycling. When we first learn to ride a bike, we have to think of every aspect of the experience because every part of it is new: keep your balance and your feet on the pedals, put pressure on the pedals to turn them, hold the handlebars, steer the bike, watch for hazards. It's all incredibly complex, takes a huge amount of concentration. But it doesn't take long before riding a bike requires little if any thought whatsoever. We no longer have to think about what we're doing because a pathway has formed and the response to those bike-riding triggers is automatic. The same is true of driving a car. Remember when you learned to drive? There were a hundred things to think about. Now consider how often you reach a destination with little awareness of how you got there–you drove on "autopilot." Driving on autopilot has certain advantages, but it's also not without hazards!

We are born with the primitive, reactive pathways that result in fight-flight-or-freeze reactions already in place. They are quick and unconscious for good reason: to instantly protect us from life-threatening danger. Conscious pathways, on the other hand, must be developed over time. Paulo had taken a step in the direction of building conscious pathways by using the suggestions from the anger management class. By counting to 10, he stopped himself from going into his usual automatic reaction pathway. (Breaking the pattern of automatic use is a critical step in developing a new pathway.) By making himself describe his intended action, he engaged the intellectual part of his brain. He put words on his intentions, rather than just staying in the helpless, angry feelings.

But Paulo recognized this was not enough. Once he was empowered to engage the more intellectual parts of his brain, he wanted to do it more. Luckily, this is possible. In fact, the way we experience the world is through thoughts about our relationship with it. These thoughts may occur so quickly that they are under our conscious radar. If an animal charges towards you, for example, you probably won't be aware that your decision to flee or not is based on your almost-instantaneous assessment of relevant information: if it's your beloved pet, you may open your arms to greet it; if it's a stranger's pit bull broken away from its leash, you'll likely choose a different response.

REWIRING THE BRAIN TO BETTER HANDLE EMOTIONS

The good news is we don't have to be prisoners of the neurological pathways we've previously laid down in our brains. Though we develop pathways to particular thoughts in response to like experiences, we also have the ability to develop new thoughts in response to those same triggers. With practice, we can train ourselves to recognize problematic thoughts and choose more beneficial ones. By doing so, we create new more productive pathways that override the old ones; they are less emotionally reactive and enable us to make better choices. The more we use the new pathways, the stronger they become. Eventually, they are more natural than the less-desired ones we replaced. Like using your left hand if you are right handed (or vice versa), it may seem unnatural, uncomfortable and clumsy at first, but with practice it can be done—it can even be done *well*. Similarly, the more you use new, positive, less-reactive pathways and choices, and the less you use the old negative assessments and reactive behaviors, the more natural and comfortable the new ways feel. This is not to say that the process of creating new pathways is easy. *Oh no! Certainly not!* It requires a lot of patience and practice. But the rewards are most definitely worth it.

Paulo recognized that although he tended to be irritable, he was not angry. His outbursts were more related to feeling helpless than being angry. Feeling helpless was Paulo's automatic reaction to certain triggers. I wondered if replacing his "I'm helpless" assessment with a more constructive empowering assessment in the face of certain triggers might be useful. It would, I thought, help him change his experience of frustrating situations and decrease some of the emotional lability he experienced. He had already shown he was able to count to 10 and evaluate his desired actions. Likewise, by examining the thoughts that led to his frustration, he could alter the feelings that caused the problem in the first place.

CHANGE YOUR THINKING TO CHANGE YOUR BEHAVIOR

How do you know if your thoughts need changing? The answer is pretty simple: by how the thoughts make you feel. This basic premise is one of the theories behind cognitive behavioral therapy (CBT), a type of psychotherapy developed by psychiatrist Aaron Beck in the 1960s. Beck believed thoughts that make us feel bad are likely "cognitive distortions." Cognitive distortions are exaggerated, irrational and often negative thoughts, which produce negatively distorted views of experiences. These distortions then generate negative feelings that lead to emotional activation and even outbursts such as those Paulo experienced.

Here's an example to illustrate the concept of how our thoughts are not attached to events, but rather to our *interpretation* of those events:

Let's say home prices are going down. There is nothing inherently negative or positive about falling house prices. Your perspective, however, may lead you to think certain thoughts about the price decline, which in turn may cause you to feel good, bad, or whatever. If you want to buy a home, you may think, "Hey, this is great, prices are going down, I can afford to buy my own place," which might make you feel happy. If, on the other hand, you want to sell the home you're in because your company has transferred you abroad, you may think: "I'm going to suffer a financial loss" which may cause you to feel bad about losing money, or angry at your company for transferring you, or. . .. you get the idea. The fact that home prices are dropping is *neutral*, it doesn't make you feel happy, sad, or angry, it's the *thought* about what the decline might mean to you, *your interpretation* of the fact, *your thought about the fact* that causes the feeling.

Paulo's lifelong experience of being unable to solve problems caused him to automatically react with frustration because he assumed he would be unable to solve *this particular problem*, which made him feel helpless, which in turn led to uncontrollable anger and the subsequent outbursts. Together Paulo and I reviewed a list of examples of cognitive distortions and found that his habit of reacting to frustration with the beliefs that we would be unable to solve the problem and the thought that we was helpless fit under the distortion known as "jumping to conclusions." On a subconscious level, if he wasn't instantly able to find a solution to a problem, Paulo jumped to the conclusion that he was helpless. His reason for doing this brought up another cognitive distortion "overgeneralization." Paulo assumed he would be unable to solve the problem because he had so many experiences of being unable to solve other problems in the past.

Paulo changed his emotional reactions step by step. First, he developed a greater awareness of his overwhelming frustration. That may sound strange, but sometimes when feelings are intense, it's hard to know exactly what it is we feel. So, the first step is to pause, identify the feeling and name it. Often just naming the feeling has a calming effect. Paulo practiced naming his feelings. When he began to feel intensely frustrated, he would stop, breathe, focus on the feeling, and verbalize what he felt: "I feel incredibly frustrated." Ironically, Paulo noticed when he said the words aloud, he immediately felt less frustrated and more in control.

The next step was to examine the thoughts that bubbled under the surface of the frustration. If he was jumping to the conclusion that he couldn't solve the problem–say, fix the computer, for example–he then asked himself if he was over-generalizing about his inability. Had he ever successfully fixed a problem on the computer? Paulo admitted he had discovered ways to fix computer issues at work–he either got help from a friend or called tech support. This realization made Paulo feel a little less helpless, which in turn helped him to feel less frustrated, and reduced the likelihood of an impulsive and counter-productive reaction such as throwing the computer against the wall.

Once he got the hang of identifying and naming his "negative" emotions, and looking at the underlying thoughts that caused them, he had another tool he could use to manage frustration and anger. Like a snowball effect, this *further* decreased his feelings of helplessness and increased his sense of control. We then looked at the rest of the cognitive distortions, some of which are listed in the cognitive distortions exercise below as well as at the end of the book. Like most of us (ADHDers *and* non-ADHDers), we found Paulo regularly made many cognitive distortions and reacted from that feeling of helplessness.

What about Jessica and her moodiness? Though her moods often came out of nowhere, she too overreacted to experiences as a result of her thoughts. If her child had trouble in school, she found herself personalizing it by assuming it was because she was a "bad mother." Rather than seeing there might be several explanations for the child's difficulty, she totally blamed herself. No wonder she was upset. When she examined and subsequently changed he cognitive distortions she greatly increased her understanding and control over the emotions that had caused a whole host of problems in her life.

Gaining an awareness of cognitive distortions and using it to change our thoughts and feelings is a powerful way for all of us (ADHDers and non-ADHDers alike) to look at life experiences in a more positive, productive and empowering light.

Now let's move on to the next two chapters, where we'll take a look at the last remaining pair of the seven symptoms manifested by adult ADHDers: inner restlessness and impulsivity.

Key Puzzle Pieces Summary

1. Cognitive distortions may negatively impact the way we see the world.

2. Identifying your emotions can help you get to the root of behaviors.

3. ADHD can be easily misdiagnosed because its symptoms are often similar to those of other diseases and disorders.

4. Pathways in our brains may cause us to act without thinking.

5. We don't have to be prisoners to our neurochemistry or existing behaviors.

Useful Exercises

BEWARE OF COGNITIVE DISTORTIONS

These top 10 "distorted" ways of thinking lead people to react to life's circumstances with negative feelings. In case you think you don't think like this, think again! We all use cognitive distortions from time to time. Problems arise when we use them to the point that our distorted view of reality makes us unhappy. Ask yourself which of the distortions listed below you have used. The more aware you are that a thought is a distortion, the more you realize you can choose a different thought—one that might make you feel better. (Adapted from Feeling Good, by David Burns, MD (New York: Avon Books, 1999, an excellent and user-friendly resource for understanding and applying cognitive therapy techniques.)

Overgeneralization: You see a single negative event as a never-ending pattern of defeat. If a bird craps on your window, you think birds are always crapping on your window, ignoring the many days they haven't.

Disqualifying the positive: You reject positive experiences by insisting they "don't count" for some reason or other. Someone giving you a compliment is "just being nice." This allows you to maintain a negative belief even if it is contradicted.

All-or-nothing thinking: You see things in black-or-white categories. For example, if your performance falls short of perfect, you see yourself as a total failure.

Mental filter: You pick out a single negative detail and dwell on it exclusively so that your vision of all reality becomes darkened, like the drop of ink that discolors an entire cup of water.

Jumping to conclusions: You make a negative interpretation even though there are no definite facts that convincingly support your conclusion. This is done through "mind reading" (assuming the motivation behind someone's actions) and "fortune telling" (assuming a negative outcome for an event).

"Catastrophizing:" You exaggerate the importance of things (such as your goof-up or someone else's achievement), or you inappropriately shrink things until they appear tiny (your own desirable qualities or another's imperfections). This is also called "the binocular trick."

Emotional reasoning: You assume your negative emotions necessarily reflect the way things really are: "I feel it, therefore it must be true." Example: Assuming you're fat because you feel fat that day.

"Should" statements: You try to motivate yourself with "should" and "shouldn't," as if you had to be whipped and punished before you could be expected to do anything. "Musts" and "oughts" are also offenders. Example: I should exercise more; I shouldn't have eaten that piece of cake.

Labeling: Instead of describing an error, you attach a label—"I'm a loser," "she's a jerk."

Personalization: You assume yourself to be responsible for an outside event. You confuse influence with control (my child got an F because I am a terrible mother).

Take Action

Train your brain to analyze your thoughts before they lead to emotional reactions. Take a few minutes to think about a difficulty you are having in life and see what cognitive distortions you can identify in your thoughts. Write a few of them here:

1. _____

2. _____

3. _____

Each day, make a point of noticing when you are using these cognitive distortions. List here what effects each statement has on your mood and how you reacted after the thought.

Situation:

_____

_____

_____

_____

_____

Cognitive distortion:

_____

_____

_____

_____

_____

(Continued)

How the thought made me feel:

_____

_____

_____

_____

_____

How I reacted:

_____

_____

_____

_____

_____

How I would like to have reacted:

_____

_____

_____

_____

_____

What thought I would need to have to lead to the more positive reaction:

_____

_____

_____

_____

_____

"UPSCALE" YOUR THOUGHTS

In the last activity, you analyzed your thoughts to see how they lead to reactions and affect your mood. Observing the connection between thoughts and moods is helpful. You may find yourself already automatically substituting unhelpful thoughts for other more positive ones.

One way to change your thoughts (and stabilize your mood) is to transform them using the "thought transformation scale." (See picture below.)

Make a scale of your thoughts from level 1 to 10, with level 1 being the kind of thought that causes you to feel distress and level 10 being the kind of thought that, if you believed it, would make you feel serene. For example, if looking at your to-do list makes you feel overwhelmed, the thought behind the feeling might be "I'll never get this done," which leads you to feel distressed. The thought "I'll never get this done" would go on the scale under level 1. A serene, level 10 thought might be "Everything will be accomplished easily and quickly."

I can almost hear your protest: "If only it were as simple as telling myself to think the level 10 thought and to feel better!" True, it's not that simple. Looking on the bright side does not immediately change your reality. It may work in the long term however—especially if you believe it! Luckily, you don't have to go from your level 1 to level 10 thought to feel better right away, here and now. You only have to train your brain to shift or lean in that positive direction. By moving away from the problematic thought and toward one that is more positive, you will actually change your neural pathways.

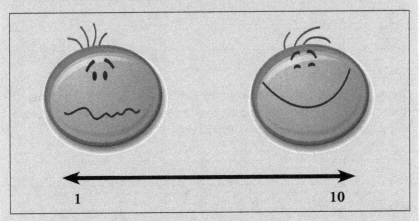

Take this in incremental steps. When you find yourself thinking in the reactionary negative perspective, consider leaning one or two steps

(Continued)

toward a more positive outlook. You want to think of the level 10 thought to know what thought you want to move towards. However, you only need to think a thought one or two levels above the one you think now to feel somewhat better. A slight shift in thought is more likely to be believable, and therefore more effective in changing your mood.

Take Action

Identify a thought that causes you to feel negatively. This could be one of the cognitive distortions you identified above.

Problem thought:

_____

_____

_____

_____

_____

Assign a number between 1 (causing distress) and 10 (leading to serenity) to the thought: _____

Identify a possible level 10 thought related to the situation:

_____

_____

_____

_____

_____

Transform your problem thought to one that is closer to the level 10 thought. The new thought doesn't need to be a 10, it just needs to be believable to make you feel somewhat better.

_____

_____

_____

_____

_____

Whenever you find yourself tempted toward a negative thought throughout the day, train your brain to instead repeat the more positive thought.
You'll be surprised by the effects!

_____Thirty Days Completed

Bravo! You're on the road to better ways of thinking!

CHAPTER 6

Inner Restlessness

INNER RESTLESSNESS: THE ADULT VERSION OF HYPERACTIVITY

Hyperactivity is less evident in adult ADHDers than it is in children with ADHD. So what happens to the hyperactivity for which ADHD kids are renowned? As ADHD has become better understood, both healthcare professionals and ADHDers themselves realize hyperactivity manifests differently in adults than it does in children—it shows up as an underlying inner restlessness.

Hyperactive behavior is easy to spot in ADHD children. They constantly fidget and are unable to sit still. They also have difficulty engaging in leisure activities quietly. As I mentioned in the overview, they are sometimes likened to the famous Energizer Bunny that just keeps on going and going. Parents often describe their ADHD children as being driven by some unseen motor that never seems to run out of fuel.

Restlessness remains in ADHD adults, but it's often subtle and therefore more difficult to detect. Adult ADHDers typically experience it as an internal sensation, which may not be noticeable to anyone but themselves. They have difficulty relaxing, and need constant stimulation to feel at ease.

Many adult ADHDers gravitate toward fields that allow for more creativity, which means they're usually more excited by, and able to focus on, their work. They also tend not to choose employment that requires them to sit all day, as they had to do as schoolchildren. As a result, ADHD adults may not exhibit as many outward symptoms of hyperactivity as ADHD children. However, their vague sense of inner restlessness, while less obvious than youthful hyperactivity, is still problematic.

The most common manifestation of inner restlessness in adult ADHDers is emotional instability. When they're active, excited and/or stimulated, they feel "up" and alive; when they're inactive, they quickly become bored, unhappy and discontent. Their mood changes are often swift and dramatic, and feel tortuous and unpredictable to the ADHDer and those around them. If you've ever been on an emotional roller coaster, you know how challenging the ups and downs are—unlike the amusement park ride, they involve more chills than thrills!

Before we look more deeply into the issues of inner restlessness in adult ADHDers, I would like to share a few words on how similar symptoms may appear in non-ADHDers exposed to high-tech stimuli from a young age.

Some researchers theorize brain development in young children may be altered by large doses of television and video games. They believe certain aspects of television, especially in children's programming, engage the brain involuntarily. You may have observed the way people tend to "zone out" while watching television. That's because it's a passive activity requiring little brain activity. As everything we do affects the brain, we should be aware that watching TV damages it by depriving it of being engaged in activities that would lead to its well-being. In fact, some researchers believe overexposure to television in young children prevents them from learning language and social skills critical for achieving higher stages of development. Besides possible deficits in academic performance, decreased development of brain areas required to consciously modulate behavior may lead to behavioral issues.[12]

Now let's go back to real-life inner restlessness in adult ADHDers.

CLASSIC CASE: KAREN

Karen, an ad agency creative director, suffered classic ADHD inner restlessness. When stimulated, she was vibrant and engaging; everyone on her team loved to be around Karen when she was "buzzing." She had loads of great ideas, and was super fun to work with, always laughing, joking and coming up with innovative ways to solve creative challenges. But when there was a dearth of new projects on which to work. . .? Watch out! Karen became a grouchy old bear. The minute her creative juices ceased flowing, she became bored and cranky. Boredom spiraled Karen down into a "funk" in which she felt she was missing out on something—not just at work, but in her whole life—though she couldn't say exactly what that something was.

Karen constantly searched for the next new thing to fire her up. She changed employers frequently, and while her brilliant campaigns had thus far kept her in high demand, her moodiness had become legendary in her industry. She worried it might soon be more difficult for her to land new jobs because of her reputation.

---

[12] Jane Healy, American Academy of Pediatrics, *AAP News*, May 1998.

When I asked Karen to describe occasions when she felt contentment, calm or inner peace, she stared at me blankly. These feelings were completely foreign to her. Karen could live in the present moment—but only if that moment fully grabbed her attention and quickened her pulse rate. The idea of just *being* in a peaceful, mindful way was something she could not recall ever having experienced. However, the realization her inner restlessness might soon become problematic to her work and career, both of which she adored, prompted her to get off the roller coaster and try the peace train instead.

INSIDE-OUT TUMBLEWEEDS?

Being mindfully aware in the present moment is a concept many people find difficult to grasp, particularly in highly developed, modern, consumer-based, accomplishment-oriented societies. Go, go, go, get, get, get, has become such an unconscious way of living we're scarcely aware of the automatons we have become. We barely pause to take a breath, let alone the time to be fully, mindfully, consciously aware of ourselves, our environment and our experiences.

People probably weren't meant to constantly be doing something—we call ourselves human "beings" after all, not human "doings." But modern life affords us opportunities to be entertained and busy all day every day without respite. What a bonanza for the inwardly restless! They don't have to look for 24/7 stimulation. All they have to do is open the door and bingo: activation city! The problem is, like an addiction, more and more stimulation is required to get the same high. Plus, negative consequences to living like this abound, not the least of which are the dramatic ups and downs of the emotional roller coaster.

There are times in our lives, such as in infancy, when we depend on others for most things. But fully functioning, healthy adults should rely in large part on themselves to fulfill their physical, emotional and spiritual needs. Instead, many of us (ADHDers and non-ADHDers alike) do the exact opposite—we look *outside* instead of *inside* of ourselves to get our needs met. Being so externally focused makes us tumbleweed-like, rolling, bouncing and being tossed about by the vagaries of whichever winds blow through our life. Not surprisingly, this leads us to feel we have no control over where we're headed or how we're going to get there.

This is especially true for ADHDers, for whom being disruptive and inattentive is a natural way of being. Many spend their lives trying to be someone other than who they naturally are (i.e. quiet, attentive, and focused) to fit in and stay out of trouble. They lose contact with themselves, and how they want to be, simply because they spend most of their lives trying to mask, change, or deny it.

This is unfortunate, because a large part of our ability to be at peace with the world and ourselves involves getting in touch with an "internal reference point" in our core being. When we focus on what goes on within us, we can more easily determine and influence our relationship with the world beyond our immediate self. "Sounds good in theory," I hear you say, but what do "internal reference points" and *being* instead of *doing* look like in reality?

Let's go back to Karen. What if Karen established a connection to the deepest aspect of her being, the place where she is grounded and content, regardless of the people, events, and circumstances around her? What if she could experience tranquility, despite the inevitable ups and downs of her external environment?

Karen related to the concept of an internal reference point by comparing it to scuba diving on the Great Barrier Reef. She had been anxious jumping off the boat as it was tossed around on the choppy sea. But once Karen descended beneath the surface turbulence, she found relative calm. At the deepest point of her dive, the fish and plants swam and swayed gently in the ocean current—it was nothing like the turbulent surface! Karen was sufficiently aware of spirituality to know others experienced similar stillness within, regardless of what occurred in their lives. She wanted to believe she also had such calm inside, but she had no idea how to find or tap into it.

MINDFULNESS: THE EXPERIENCE OF CALM AWARENESS

Luckily, there are ways to be in the present moment and experience inner calm instead of restlessness—it's simply a matter of learning and practicing them. The more one practices such techniques, the more one experiences joy in small things and feels overall contentment in life. One of the accessible skills is mindfulness, a calm experience of one's body, feelings, and thoughts: an awareness of being aware.

Being mindful is living in and experiencing the present moment without distraction. It's the practice of paying attention to your present emotions, thoughts, and body sensations without judging or reacting to them. The goal is to be less reactive and more accepting, and thus to achieve calm and inner stillness. If Karen noticed her boredom and examined it with curiosity, for example, she might be able to prevent herself from going into a funk. Also, if she noticed it *deeply*, she might even feel less bored.

Karen began her mindfulness practice with two minutes each day during which she calmly observed her breath as it went in and out. After a week of doing this when she first got to work, she noticed she started her day from a calmer and more grounded place. In fact, she enjoyed it so much she had doubled her practice time by the end of the week. Occasionally, she also remembered to breathe mindfully during the day when she felt stressed. Karen noticed that thoughts of things she had to do, or conversations she'd planned to have, occasionally "appeared" in her mind. She also sometimes dropped the practice to do something else or realized she had been daydreaming rather than consciously focusing on her breath. Nevertheless, Karen immediately saw the benefits of the practice and readily agreed to learn more.

During week two, she continued her early morning breathing exercise, but now she set the timer on her phone for five minutes instead of two. With her eyes closed, she "watched" her breath and tried to engage her other senses concurrently. She noticed, for example, the smells in the room (mostly her skinny latte with extra foam and cinnamon!), and the sounds of her co-workers as they arrived and settled into their workspaces.

I anticipated Karen would experience more "intrusive" thoughts during week two, and so it was. The explanation for this is simple. When we take something fresh and new and make it routine, it is less novel and interesting, and thus more of a focus challenge, particularly for an ADHDer. Karen assured me she would block such thoughts. The problem, I explained to Karen, is energy devoted to blocking thoughts is energy not going to noticing current sensations. In addition, when we think about our thoughts we are "in our heads," and less able to appreciate the present moment. For the most part, thoughts relate to something, which has already happened or will happen, rather than what is happening at the time.

Fortunately, intrusive thoughts can help rather than hinder mindfulness practice. Such thoughts are problematic only if the practitioner allows them to take her out of her body (and the present moment), and into her head instead. I encouraged Karen to notice thoughts as they arose, mentally label each one as "a thought," then let it go and refocus her attention on her breath and sensations. The thoughts would then become "triggers" to a more deeply mindful state of consciousness. They would be clouds in the sky of her breathing practice, drifting on the surface of the deeper space of her mind and body. The key is to not "judge" the thoughts or examine them too much–it's best just to let them swim through your consciousness like sunfish through a coral reef. In this way, you leave behind the superficial "choppiness" of life to reach the stillness that lies on the ocean floor of your being.

THE EMOTIONAL ROLLER COASTER

Karen saw how this practice would help her be more centered and less reactive, but didn't think it would alleviate the ups and downs of the emotional roller coaster. She didn't know the degree to which her thoughts had an emotional effect on her. If a thought involved the need to do something, she barely perceived the anxiety accompanying it; she went right into the reactionary mode of either doing something or thinking about what she needed to do. It was so habitual she didn't realize the reactions had occurred or that they were connected to her thoughts. If she allowed her brain to continue processing thoughts in this way, she would remain vulnerable to the emotional responses it induced. The only way off the roller coaster was to process her thoughts differently, which was what she learned to do through the mindfulness practice.

To help Karen understand how profound mindfulness can be, I shared some research showing how getting the brain to work differently creates new connections and pathways among its cells and neurons, and leads to new ways of experiencing the world. A recent study published in the journal Psychological Science[13] demonstrates how this occurs with mindfulness practice.

Researchers put subjects into a brain scanner that showed which parts of the subjects' brains responded to a series of photographs. The photographs were like thoughts—popping into the subjects' awareness so fast they had time only to react, not to think. When the photographs depicted images/stimuli characterized as "angry" or "fearful," the instinctual parts of the subjects' brains were activated.

The subjects then practiced mindfulness for several weeks. Whenever they experienced anger or fear, they were asked to notice and label it; thus: "This is anger," or "This is fear."

The researchers then repeated the brain scans using the same photographs. This time, another area of the brain responded–the higher-ordered, observing part, where information is taken in and processed before it's acted upon. Instead of experiencing a fast, thoughtless reaction when exposed to the angry and/or fearful stimuli, the subjects' brains now took a step back and processed the visual information in a new way. The research helped Karen understand how mindfulness could help her get off the emotional roller coaster:

---

[13] Lieberman, M. D., Eisengerger, N. I., Crockett, M. J., Tom, S. M., Pfeifer, J. H., & Way, B. M., "Putting feelings into words: Affect labeling disrupts amygdala activity in response to affective stimuli," *Psychological Science*, (2007) 18(5), 421-428.

by observing her thoughts, rather than reacting to them, she would be better able to remain calm, regardless of what happened in her life.

FIGHT, FLIGHT, FREEZE

As Karen learned to relax her mind, she became more aware of tension in her body. All of her *doing* left little time for *being*—she rarely relaxed. A life of constant reactivity resulted in constant tension, which became worse when she felt stressed. As we've already seen, all human beings react to life-threatening situations with a physical response known as "fight, flight, or freeze; it's a healthy and sometimes necessary part of functioning, as a real-life surfing experience of my own clearly demonstrates.

It was a beautiful day, and I was alone on the ocean (or so I thought) enjoying my pick of the incoming waves. Suddenly, I had company—a five-foot-long shark swam under my surfboard! At first, I thought it was kind of cool. I love to see harmless sharks when I scuba dive, and this one appeared to be one of those.

I was about to go for another wave when I noticed my new friend had circled around to take another look at me. That was odd. In fact, he appeared to be stopped, hovering a few feet away, just watching me. I began to feel uncomfortable. "Friendly" sharks don't tend to hang out and "stare" like that. He made another circle around me, returned to the same spot and hovered once again. Now I felt more than just uncomfortable. I was terrified, and in full fight, flight, or freeze mode. So, what did I do?

I wish I could impress you with my valor, but engaging the shark never crossed my mind. And, though I certainly wanted to flee to the beach, making sudden moves when it was obviously watching me seemed ill advised. Instead, I froze: ever so slowly, with extreme caution, I pulled my arms and legs onto the board. . .and waited. I barely moved, hardly daring to even breathe, until the shark lost interest, turned tail and swam off, at which point I rode the next wave into shore.

My close encounter with "jaws" is a good example of when the fight, flight, or freeze response is useful; but having it unnecessarily and repeatedly activated is problematic. Fight, flight or freeze is great for occasional high stress situations—it's what keeps us safe when we are in danger. Unfortunately, when it's engaged too frequently (or worse, chronically), it adversely affects our bodies. In general, the daily stressors we experience are neither "fightable" nor "flee-able," so many of us tend to freeze in response—we go from the stressful commute, to the stressful job, to the stressful home life in a "frozen" state.

That was Karen: her muscles tense and frozen into position, her shoulders perpetually up to her ears. When she was about to speak with someone, she would often brace herself, further tensing, without even knowing it.

KAREN LEARNS TO CHILLAX EVEN MORE. . .

Karen knew she was perpetually tense, but did little to rid herself of the tension–until we met. I suggested to her that she would be less tense and more productive at work if she relaxed when away from the office. This idea interested her, for obvious reasons. She didn't see any value in holding tension, and was willing to try anything to feel less tired and worn out. Once she had successfully implemented being more mindful, I suggested she take two more steps: 1) focus intensely on her breathing, and 2) learn to relax her muscles.

During one of our sessions, I asked her to close her eyes and breathe in deeply through her nose, and, on the first breath, let her abdomen fill with air; the second breath she expanded into her chest, to the point she felt her ribs push apart. After only two deep breaths, she felt much calmer. She could not remember the last time she had breathed so deeply, and felt so relaxed. That's because Karen did what most of us do when we're locked in the "freeze" response: we breathe shallowly into our chest. We get enough air to carry on, but miss the greater energy resulting from a thorough intake of oxygen and exhalation of waste.

Next we worked on her muscle tension. Karen's body had learned to hold itself in a tense, stiff way; she had to *teach* it to relax. But first she had to notice when and where in her body she held tension. Just as taking deep breaths allowed her to experience how shallow her normal breathing was, a relaxation exercise put her in touch with how tense her muscles were.

For the next week, Karen took a few minutes to practice relaxation after work. She got into a comfortable position, closed her eyes and breathed deeply; she imagined the air going to each part of her body, starting with her toes and moving up, as she relaxed one part after another. As she alternated between tensing and relaxing she became aware of how different relaxation felt from tension. After several days of practice, she could identify when she started to tense during the day. She would then exaggerate tensing her muscles and then relax them. This practice decreased some of the anxiety that provoked her tension, and gave her an effective way to relax whenever she felt herself becoming tense. All of a sudden work became much less stressful!

Being mindful and learning to relax can be wonderfully liberating practices for anyone–ADHDers and non-ADHDers alike. Start using these techniques today, and I guarantee you will see the world from a whole new perspective.

Key Puzzle Pieces Summary

1. Hyperactivity manifests as inner restlessness in ADHD adults. Inner restlessness often shows up as emotional instability.

2. Go, go, go, get, get, get has become an unconscious way of living for both ADHDers and non-ADHDers alike.

3. Peace and calm are found inside (not outside) ourselves. Being mindful helps us access the calmness at our core.

4. Fight, flight and freeze are predictable, protective, and natural reactions to external threats.

5. Breathe deeply with intention, and observe how the practice changes your world.

Useful Exercises

BREATHE INTO RELAXATION WITH PRANAYAMA

This breathing exercise is based on one of the ancient yogic practices of pranayama. "Prana" is Sanskrit for life force, and "yama" refers to action. So, it is an action of the life force, pranayama draws the life force in and engages it. There are many different types of pranayama exercises; my favorite is alternate nostril breathing, which focuses on the breath while balancing breathing between the two nostrils.

The hands are held in what is called a "mudra." The idea of a mudra is to lock in the sensation or benefits of a practice. The theory is, with time, you can capture the benefits so well within the mudra that, eventually, placing the hands in the mudra alone will give the benefits of the practice. The mudra for alternate nostril breathing is to fold the first two fingers of the right hand downwards toward the palm. The interesting thing about this position is that the fingers are touching at what is called the "lung point" in Chinese medicine.

- The left hand is held with the tip of the thumb and first finger pressed together and resting on the knee. Close your eyes and get ready to relax.
- Using the thumb of the right hand, press the right nostril closed and take a deep breath in through the left nostril. This is usually done to a count of four (see the first photo on next page).
- After counting to four, close both nostrils by bringing the pinky and ring finger of the right hand to press against the left nostril. Hold your breath in this position for a count of sixteen (see the middle photo on next page).
- At the end of sixteen seconds, release the thumb from the right nostril and breathe out to a count of eight seconds (see the last photo on next page).
- Continue to do this process by then leaving the thumb off of the right nostril so that it can breathe in.
- Hold both nostrils again and then release the left nostril to breathe out.
- Breathe in through the left nostril, hold, and breathe out through the right.

- Breathe in through the right nostril, hold, and breathe out through the left.
- Continue to do this for nine rounds.

Doing the four-sixteen-eight count may be hard at first, so I suggest start with two-eight-four; the proportions are the same, and you will incur a similar benefit. Practice once daily.

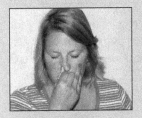 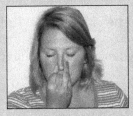 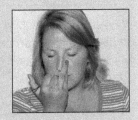

Take Action

Choose a time each day when you feel the greatest need to relax. It could be when you drive, before work, after work, even during work! Record it here. The time I most need, and can reliably complete, a session of this breathing exercise is:

_____

_____

_____

_____

_____

Things that may possibly get in the way of doing this exercise daily:

_____

_____

_____

_____

(Continued)

How I will manage these:

_____

_____

_____

_____

_____

Place a check mark here when you've done this practice once per day for 30 days in a row (don't worry if you miss a day and have to start over; just keep looking at what is getting in the way and continue until you achieve 30 consecutive days).

_____Thirty Days Completed!

Take a deep breath of congratulations!

USE MINDFULNESS TO BE MORE AWARE

This mindfulness practice involves eating. I like to use a raisin to demonstrate this, but other foods work equally well. The objective is to engage each of your senses in order to fully experience a particular activity. Start by looking at the raisin closely. Spend at least one minute looking at it like you've never seen one before. Notice the way the light hits it, the various grooves, any variation in color.

Next, engage your sense of smell. Hold it up to your nose and notice if there is a smell that you might not have been aware of previously.

Now, use the sense of touch. Spend another minute moving the raisin around in your fingers. Notice the consistency as you squeeze it slightly and run your fingers over the grooves.

Then, put the raisin in your mouth and feel those same grooves with the tongue, moving it around in the mouth for a while to really feel it before starting to chew. When you're ready to take a bite, notice the taste difference between how it tasted before and after biting into it. Notice as much as possible about the taste of the raisin; think of words to describe it. Savor the taste for as long as you can before you swallow it.

Now, incorporate such mindfulness into all areas of your life—notice when you are out of the present moment and engage your senses to get back into it. As you practice, you will become more adept at recognizing when you are out of your deep, still center. Do this daily, regardless of what is going on in your life. You will eventually realize there is a part of you, underneath everything else, that is unaffected by the turbulence of daily life, and you will experience life from a place of greater equanimity.

Take Action

Describe your experience of doing this exercise so that you will remember its benefits and be motivated to do it again:

_____

_____

_____

_____

_____

(Continued)

List an experience that you could use for five minutes each day to engage your senses fully. For example, you could use the eating exercise described above, or simply choose moments to observe and experience the environment around and within you.

_____

_____

_____

_____

_____

Place a mark here when you have completed 30 days in a row of doing five minutes of mindfulness each day.

_____Thirty Days Completed!

Kudos on being more mindful!

RELAX EACH AND EVERY PART OF YOU

The first step towards relaxation is to feel the difference between relaxation and tension. This exercise helps you do it. You may want to read through the exercise a few times until you can follow it without looking; alternatively, have someone read it to you. Start by slowly taking a few deep breaths in through the nose and imagine the breath filling first the abdomen and then each part of the body. Do this until you start to feel any tension fade. If it helps, give the breath a color, like golden yellow, and then imagine filling each part of your body with the color. Picturing the body helps to engage parts of your brain not involved with thinking, and gives your thinking mind a break. When you are ready, slowly tense and release each part of your body, starting with your toes and going all of the way up to each part of your face. By tensing and then releasing each part, one at a time, you feel the difference between tension and relaxation as the muscles release. Continue to do this until all of the muscles in your body have been tensed and released.

Continue to breathe and enjoy the relaxation for as long as you want, or allow yourself to drift off into sleep. When you are ready to come out of this relaxed state, slowly wiggle your fingers and toes and then roll your arms and legs, feeling energy returning to each part of your body before getting up slowly.

Remember how this relaxation feels and bring yourself back to it whenever you feel tension rising in your body.

Take Action

Describe how this relaxation exercise made you feel:

_____

_____

_____

_____

_____

Choose a time each day when you can set aside at least five minutes to do this exercise. Just before sleep might be a good choice.

_____

(Continued)

After you have done this exercise for five minutes for 30 days in a row, make a mark here.

_____Thirty Days Completed.

Bravo!

Describe any benefits you noticed over the 30 days. This will make you more likely to make the practice a lifetime habit.

_____

_____

_____

_____

_____

CHAPTER 7

Impulsivity

Impulsive Behavior: Do It NOW if Not Sooner!

Impulsivity, the final on our list of seven symptoms, is easy to spot in ADHD children: they leave their seats, talk excessively, are unable to wait in a line, and feel compelled to touch and explore everything they see. But how does it manifest in ADHD adults?

Many Adult ADHDers manage to avoid situations where they are forced to stay in one place all day. They may have a lot of difficulty waiting in line, but have likely figured out they must, due to the consequences of not doing so. Likewise, they've probably learned to keep their hands to themselves, rather than touching and exploring everything in their environment.

In ADHD adults, impulsivity typically involves making snap decisions rather than taking the time to examine pertinent details. They may be quite reckless, and are prone to engaging in risky behaviors such as substance abuse, shoplifting, and others. Impulsivity also manifests as statements blurted out without any thought of their potential impact. As we saw in Chapter 4 (Social Issues), this affects ADHDers' abilities to communicate effectively. Impulsive ADHDers may also switch rapidly from one task to another, because their interest in individual tasks quickly wanes, or they feel uncomfortable if new ideas aren't acted on immediately.

From the child who can't keep from grabbing what he or she wants to the adult who can't filter what he or she says, being uncontrollably impulsive devastates the lives of ADHDers of all ages. Because impulsivity may be expressed both verbally and in actions, it plays a role in all kinds of aberrant behavior, which may explain why ADHDers seem disproportionately to suffer negative consequences such as arrests, divorces, accidents, and the like. Non-ADHDers who exhibit the same kinds of impulsive behaviors suffer similar impacts.

As I have said many times in previous chapters, the nature of our technological society causes non-ADHDers to experience ADHD-like symptoms.

So it is with impulsive behavior. The constant bombardment of technology and information may cause non-ADHDers to also be more impulsive, distracted and unable to concentrate. With so many bits of information available simultaneously through e-mail, digital devices, TV, and our surroundings, we're almost forced to multitask. To attend to a multitude of stimuli at once, the brain shifts rapidly between various types of information and activities. Research shows, over time, the shifting strengthens the brain's capacity to leave one task for another. That's why multitasking seems easier with practice. In fact, we become so accustomed to doing it, we forget how to focus without distractions. However, by learning to shift focus rapidly, we may become less able to concentrate, particularly when we deal with problems requiring time and reflection. The result is people *without* ADHD are behaving more like people *with* ADHD, as their brains become "trained" to function in more reactive and restless ways.[14]

To get a better understanding of impulsive behavior in ADHDers, let's visit with Marie and Antonio.

MARIE TAKES IT TO THE LIMIT, AND BEYOND

Marie was highly impulsive, and had been off and on ADHD medications from a relatively young age. Though she was an honest and moral person, Marie had stolen from shops and stores as a teenager. Frustrated by the fact that her parents didn't want her to be too flashy and wouldn't let her wear makeup and jewelry in junior high, she shoplifted things she wanted, but was forbidden by her parents to have. She knew it was wrong, but she couldn't resist. Unlike many shoplifters, Marie didn't get a thrill from stealing. She did it because she couldn't come up with other options for getting what she wanted. As she grew older and had more money, the shoplifting stopped, but other problems started.

Driving, in particular, was a challenge. She knew the speed limits, but was unable to stick to them. She always felt the need to be somewhere *right now* (if not before!), even if there was plenty of time to reach her destination on schedule. She felt compelled to pass other vehicles regardless of their speed, because she couldn't tolerate having another car in front of her. The constant rush coupled with her lack of attention to detail resulted in a host of bumps and scrapes on her car, inflicted mostly while she tried to park in a hurry.

---

[14] Gary Small, MD, "Don't let computer use harm your brain," special from *Bottom Line/Health*, May 1, 2009.

Her driving ultimately gave Marie the impetus to stay on her ADHD medication. She didn't feel she drove any differently, but the evidence was irrefutable: when she took her medication, other drivers honked at her less. She dismissed feedback from people who said she was easier to be around when she took medication, but it was hard to ignore the clear evidence of the strangers' honking. When she committed to taking medication regularly, the driving issues (and bothersome honking) ceased.

If It's New, I've Gotta' Try It!

Antonio never understood why he'd had trouble with substance abuse in high school. It wasn't peer pressure—Antonio didn't care what others thought of him. He did his own thing, and paid no attention to the actions or reactions of those around him. He didn't consume alcohol or drugs to be cool, because he didn't care about being cool—he drank because he felt like it. But somehow he would have finished his fifth drink before he even realized he'd had the first four. He'd try any drug—the effect (slow down, speed up) didn't really matter to Antonio. The novelty of trying something new and different drove his compulsive experimentation. He couldn't resist popping the latest pill or slamming back the newest shooter. He didn't give alcohol and drug abuse a second thought, neither did he pause to think of the consequences of his behavior.

Besides specific actions such as these, being impulsive can develop into a way of life in which even major decisions are made without deliberation. Snap decisions and judgments are the order of the day. Accustomed to thinking at lightning speed and doing everything on the spur of the moment, ADHDers may assume, on some level, they have all of the required information so there's no need to further research or contemplate additional possibilities.

Likewise, lack of focus may prevent an ADHDer from assimilating additional data and leads her to make decisions with the information at hand (plus, it's easier than gathering more data!). When something is enticing, the impulse to act, coupled with the tendency to make snap decisions results in an inability to hold back—an irresistible cocktail of impulsivity. ADHDers often feel extreme discomfort when forced to wait for something; denying themselves the object or action of their desire is almost unthinkable.

"Hey, wait a minute. No one likes to wait or be denied something pleasurable, not just people with ADHD!" I hear you and a chorus of other readers chiming in. . .and once again, you're right. This type of impulsive behavior is not confined to ADHDers. Many non-ADHDers are also impulsive, particularly teenagers. In all honesty, *everyone* and *anyone* can be impulsive now and again. But most people learn the downside of being too impulsive too often because there's often hell to pay when impulsivity takes over. ADHDers, on the other hand, don't seem to learn from the consequences. Why is that? Yes, you're right again! It all comes back, as we have already seen elsewhere, to the brain.

IT'S ALL ABOUT DEVELOPMENT

Impulses can be triggered by different neurological mechanisms. Think of advertising as an example of how we react to certain stimuli. Advertisers highlight product features to entice consumers to buy goods on impulse–food ads showing people feeling good, and use words about smells and taste, for example. Advertisers also appeal to the subconscious to boost sales. Think of the word "mouthwatering." Does it produce any physical reaction when you do? Are you starting to salivate? Perhaps you are reminded you haven't eaten anything in the last few hours and you're beginning to feel hungry? Isn't the power of suggestion an amazing thing? Maybe you even want to get up and get something to eat right now, but you are resisting the impulse, because you want to finish this chapter.

Luckily, impulses generated by advertising are dealt with primarily by the "intellectual" part of the brain; it processes the information that allows us to decide whether or not to act. Something may appeal to us on a primitive level, but the higher-ordered part of the brain processes the desire and evaluates it along with other information, such as safety and laws, before taking action. For this to work effectively, we must have relevant information, as well as the ability to examine our impulses before we act. Babies automatically put things in their mouths, because they don't know what's edible and what's not. Even if they did, their infant brains are not sufficiently developed to process such information: signals don't get beyond the primitive brain because the pathways to the higher-ordered, thinking part of the brain are not yet developed. The pathways themselves are there, but not in a usable state. Before they can be used, they must be coated with *myelin* (in a process called "myelination"), which allows information to be more easily transmitted from one part of the brain to another–much like electrical wires are coated to allow the effective transmission of electricity.

Myelination does not occur in the higher-ordered, frontal part of the brain until late adolescence or early adulthood. This partly explains the propensity of teenagers to engage in high-risk behaviors, even when cognizant of the potentially tragic consequences. Modern-day examples of crazy stunts include "car surfing" and "ghost riding" in which daredevils "surf" on the hoods of moving vehicles, and/or drag beside or behind the vehicles in carts or on skateboards. The results can be fatal. Though the information about safety issues may be in the teen brain, it's not readily available when an impulse arises because the transmittal pathways are not sufficiently developed to get the data to a place where it can be properly processed. Instead (in basic terms), when she becomes excited and engaged in potentially dangerous behavior, the teen uses the primitive brain (as a kind of back-up as it were), which is not nearly as "sensible" as the higher-ordered part of the brain. The result? Impulsive behavior in which a more developed brain would certainly be less prone to engage.

ONCE UPON A SATURDAY WITH AN IMPULSIVE ADHD BRAIN

Now let's take a look at the ADHD brain. It would be overly simplistic to describe it as "teenaged," though it can certainly feel like it to the ADHDer and look like it to observers! ADHD brains undergo the usual stages of maturation. However, ADHDers don't have easy access to the higher-ordered, intellectual parts of their brains. Why not? Because the neurons in the higher-ordered part of ADHD brains process neurochemicals ineffectively. Fortunately, proper brain functioning can be induced with treatment to increase the level of neurochemicals, and compensate for deficient processing.

On the other hand, treatment is not a cure-all. Just like everybody else, ADHDers develop ways of behaving over many years. Though the neurochemistry can change right away, modifying deeply entrenched behavior patterns may prove challenging, even when modification is facilitated with medication.

Like many of my patients, Antonio found medication helped him reduce the number of times he asked himself ruefully why he had said or done something silly, stupid or inappropriate. When he was properly medicated he felt less compelled to act on anything and everything presented to him. Without medication, it would seem absolutely impossible to allow something to pass him by; with medication he was able to think through benefits and consequences and make reasonable decisions before he acted, instead of regretting his actions afterward. Nevertheless, Antonio's impulsive streak remained, lurking somewhere beneath the surface. He could stop, reflect and talk himself out of doing something dangerous, but he wondered if impulsivity might lie behind numerous projects that languished about his home in various stages of completion. He started all kinds of things, but rarely finished.

In one session, Antonio described to me this sequence of events from the previous Saturday:

"I decided I really should get going on building the new bar I had planned for the downstairs room I wanted to renovate. I jotted down a few of the things I thought I would need then headed to the hardware store. On the way, I remembered I had to go to the pharmacy to pick up my meds, and dashed in really quickly to get them. While I was there, I ran into Jack. I told him I was on my way to the hardware store to get stuff for the bar project which prompted him to tell me about his latest reno–a new patio. It sounded really cool, so I stopped to take a look at it. When I saw the patio, I thought, hey, I should build one of these too, and since I was going to be at the hardware store anyway, I might as well get supplies to build an outdoor patio as well as the basement bar. I got everything I thought I needed at the store and then headed home.

I started right in on the bar when I got back, but it wasn't long before I felt hungry, so I stopped for a snack. While I was in the kitchen, I noticed there were a couple of days' worth of un-opened mail on the counter, so I started to go through it. When I came to a bill from the landscaping company, it made me think about the patio project and I wondered if I had got all the stuff I needed. So I left the mail and went out back where I had dumped the supplies. I spread everything out to see if I was missing any-thing. . . I realized I had forgotten a couple of key things, so I popped back to the hardware store. By the time I got back it was getting close to dinner, I was tired, and basically nothing had got done. There was a pile of half-opened mail on the kitchen counter, stuff spread all over the back yard, tools everywhere in the base-ment where I had started to work on the bar. . .."

Antonio sighed deeply, and looked at me in despair. "Why can't I ever seem to get anything done?" he asked, frustration clearly evident in his voice.

One might be tempted to attribute Antonio's problems completing projects with an inability to follow through (the ADHD symptom we cov-ered in Chapter 2). But Antonio was right to wonder if it might be due to impulsivity. He didn't become bored or overwhelmed with his tasks, which is usually what happens with ADHDers who have follow-through issues. There just always seemed to be one more thing to which he should quickly attend before he got back to the other thing (or things) he had already begun. Like his experiences with substance abuse, he was almost unaware he was doing something until he was already far into it. He knew he should complete one task before starting another, but it didn't make sense to him to put things off. It just seemed easier and more sensible to get them done in the moment. When spontaneous opportunities arose, such as running into the friend with the freshly built patio, why not take advantage of them? And, wasn't it more efficient to pop into the pharmacy on the way to somewhere else than to make a separate trip?

Antonio's thoughts on opportunities and efficiency made sense, but something had to change or he would continue to be frustrated by his home full of unfinished projects. I asked him to imagine his Saturday reconstructed: what if he'd gone straight to the hardware store and back home, worked on his project, completed it, dealt with the mail, gone to see his friend's patio, stopped by the pharmacy, and started his own patio project. Antonio took a deep breath and allowed himself to access his imagination. As he did, he began to feel anxious. No, he absolutely could not stay on one task. He might forget all about doing the other tasks and miss out.

ANTONIO TAKES CONTROL

As an experiment, Antonio agreed to complete one task before going on to another for one week. To decrease his anxiety, he would put other ideas that occurred to him on a list, so he could continue his primary task knowing nothing would be forgotten. Though the impulses would still arise and he would be uncomfortable putting them aside, it was much easier to do so knowing he would come back to them later.

When he made these lists, Antonio noticed how quickly they filled up with things to do. It became obvious he could not possibly complete all the tasks within the time he had available. Once he saw them listed, he also quickly recognized one way to manage the tasks and projects was to choose which ones he really wanted to do, or that had to be done, and prioritize them. When he reviewed his Saturday for example, he realized he would prefer to sort the mail, go to the pharmacy and finish the bar project, rather than see his friend's patio and start on a new patio project.

All of a sudden he was *choosing* one thing over another rather than missing out. Making a conscious choice put a whole new spin on things! Antonio began to feel more in control and less driven by the need to be a part of anything and everything that randomly occurred at any given time. He discovered he could evaluate his choices based on what they would *bring to him*, rather than worrying about what he might *miss*. This new perspective turned things around in a way that made Antonio feel empowered and in control, rather than buffeted about by all the unfinished stuff in his life.

Another way to make sure you keep on track is to create goals and work towards them. Without a goal in mind, it is easy to become distracted and impulsively act on other "opportunities" that come along. Having goals makes it easier to evaluate particular opportunities. You can then to say "no" to opportunities which may be interesting, but which do not help you to achieve your goals, and "yes" to those you feel will be truly helpful.

We're done! Impulsivity is the final of the seven symptoms. Do you remember the other six? Decreased focus, lack of follow-through, disorganization, social issues, emotional reactivity, and inner restlessness. The remaining parts of the book comprise a conclusion, as well as appendices on treatment options, the useful exercises from each chapter, references and resources.

Key Puzzle Pieces Summary

1. In ADHD adults, impulsivity typically involves making snap decisions rather than taking the time to examine pertinent details.

2. Impulsive behavior is not confined to ADHDers; it can be triggered by different neurological mechanisms.

3. Medication can be effective in treating impulsivity, particularly if it is combined with behavioral modification techniques and strategies.

4. Writing ideas and tasks down rather than immediately acting on them is one way to become less impulsive.

5. Making conscious choices helps you remain in control.

Useful Exercises

List Your Great Ideas

One way to decrease the temptation to go off track when an idea occurs to you is to make a "Great Ideas" list. When an opportunity arises or an idea comes to you, it can be hard to not act on it right away. This may be due to impulsivity, the fear of forgetting it, or a general fear that you'll miss out if you don't jump on things immediately. To stop getting sidetracked, commit to completing one task before taking on any other.

Because it may be difficult to overcome the habit of switching between tasks, start by completing one task each day. Perhaps you've decided to read some articles for work, for example. Do that task without doing anything else until you're done. If something else that needs to be done occurs to you, write it down. When the one task is complete, notice if you still feel the need to do the others on your list. If not, don't do them; if so, try doing them one at a time as well.

Take Action

Choose one task and do it without allowing yourself to be sidetracked until it is complete:

_____

_____

Keep a list of other ideas that occur to you, and put them off until your task is done.

_____

_____

_____

_____

_____

_____

_____

_____

_____

(Continued)

_____

_____

What did you notice from doing a task this way?

_____

_____

Mark here when you've completed one task without being sidetracked each day for 30 days.

_____Complete

_____Complete

_____Complete

_____Complete

_____Complete

_____Complete

_____Complete

_____Complete

_____Complete

I bet you have a great list of great ideas. . .

Do What Works

One of the most difficult aspects of impulsivity is the frustration of not being able to do or get what you want. It's easier to tolerate, and even dissipate the frustration if you shift your focus from the experiencing the impulses to engaging the intellectual part of the brain by evaluating the situation from a different angle. One way to do this is to examine your thoughts from the perspective of "doing what works." This isn't denying what you desire, but rather incorporating additional information about your goal into your thoughts. Retrain your brain by evaluating one frustration in this way each day for 30 days using the following exercise.

Take Action

Identify one frustration you currently experience that you can do nothing about. Notice what thought about the experience is unhelpful (i.e. either makes you feel worse or involves an action with detrimental effects).

Unhelpful thought: (Example: I don't want to go to work)

_____

_____

_____

Make that thought more helpful with the following statements:

It is true that (same unhelpful thought):

_____

_____

_____

and, at the same time (positive statement that is also true):

_____

_____

Given that (same unhelpful thought),

_____

(Continued)

What do I want to do, for example, with this day, situation, etc. (For example, focus on how happy it makes me to see the check deposited into my bank account and know that I'm working towards that)

_____

_____

_____

*Do one of the following 5-minute meditations and then record whatever you experience.

1) Imagine how someone who is "calm and in control" would act in the same situation.

2) Get in touch with every aspect of the situation that is going favorably and express appreciation, in your mind, to whatever you feel to be responsible for this. (e.g. I appreciate my savings are growing, thanks to my work). This will help to keep you motivated through inevitable frustrations.

_____

_____

_____

_____

_____

_____

DEFINE & WORK TOWARDS GOALS

One way to manage impulses is to have a goal. By defining and working towards a goal, you can achieve what you desire in the long term, regardless of how many times you are sidetracked along the way. Research shows people who work towards defined goals are happier than those who do not. This is due to the way the brain engages in the process of getting to the goal, more than the achievement of the goal itself.

Think of something you want to learn, accomplish, or do; it should be something you can begin within the next month. Maybe you've always wanted to learn another language, or a dance style; perhaps you want to create a scrapbook or write a book. Create one goal for this month, then lay out the steps you will take towards achieving it.

Unlike a business plan or something you *should* do, this goal is something you want to do just because it interests you. It doesn't matter how much is accomplished by the end of the month. The point of the exercise is to observe the process to see whether setting goals and working towards them decreases the negative consequences of impulsivity and increases your happiness.

Let's say you chose to begin to learn Japanese. (Learning a language is a good choice because there is always something more that can be achieved.) Using a calendar, break your goal for the month into smaller steps. Maybe you will learn a certain number of words each day, attend a certain number of classes over the month, do something each week, etc. Depending on what feels right to you, create steps and set target dates for accomplishing the steps during the month. Now, start working towards the goal, and notice how you feel during the various parts of the process. Remember it may be easier and feel more pleasurable to watch TV or do nothing, but happiness will come from engaging your brain towards achieving something.

Take Action

Choose a goal that is important to you, and about which you will feel good achieving. Write steps you can take towards this goal, and do them for the remainder of the month. Remember the most important part of this exercise is to observe the process.

My goal is:

_____

(Continued)

To work towards this goal, I will:

_____

_____

_____

What I observed about this process was (e.g. how motivated I stayed, how important it felt, the energy I sustained towards reaching it):

_____

_____

_____

Congratulations on having set a goal and taken steps toward achieving it.

Conclusion

WHERE DO I GO FROM HERE?

I hope you now have a better understanding of ADHD, and the ways in which modern life can lead to ADHD-like symptoms in non-ADHDers. Regardless of the cause of your symptoms, the exercises in this book can help you rewire your brain from one that is "affected" to one that is *effective*. Do more than read the exercises. *Do them*. I promise they will make a difference for you, just as they did for me. When you apply the principles and do the exercises, I am 100 percent certain you will experience the power you have to rewire your brain. You can transform it from the one you have, to the one you want.

At this point, you may ask yourself: "Where do I go from here?" The answer depends on your condition. This book was designed to help you better understand yourself and your behavior, and to give you strategies and tools to help you to change if you wish. For many, reading this book and acting on the information and suggestions it contains may be enough. Others may need or want more.

ADHDers may find the benefits of the exercises difficult to appreciate without the assistance of other treatment, such as medication. If you suspect that might be the case for you, I encourage you to read the appendix on treatment options. It will help you understand what medications are available and then determine, with appropriate professional advice, which will work best for you. Remember: treatment options change constantly, and what was true at the time this book was published may no longer apply when you read it. I can't emphasize enough that this book is meant to be a *starting point* for further discussion with a certified professional. In addition, medication treatment should not be used *instead of* the exercises I have suggested, but rather *in conjunction* with them. If you choose to use medication, I encourage you to return to this book and try the exercises after you have been stabilized through

93

treatment. You should realize more profound benefits doing the exercises in tandem with treatment.

Even non-ADHDers who struggle with distraction and disorganization may require additional assistance to fully implement the strategies outlined in the previous chapters. For those who require additional personalized guidance (whether you have ADHD or not), I recommend working individually with a properly trained professional: a psychiatrist who specializes in this area, someone trained in psychotherapy, or an ADHD coach. An ADHD coach can help you set personal life goals, and guide you in achieving them.

Many people prefer to work with someone such as myself, who is an expert in all three areas. I blend the psychiatric, psychotherapeutic, and coaching modalities based on individual needs. As a thank you for purchasing this book, I am pleased to offer you an introductory session at half the usual cost. It's easy to take advantage of the special fee discount; just go to www. SciencefortheJourney.com, click on "sign up for individual sessions," and type in: *From Scattered to Centered*. You will automatically receive a 50 percent discount on your first session with me.

As with anything we want to change in life, the results of therapy and coaching are generally realized as part of a journey, rather than as an instantaneous success. Each step we take brings us closer to the person we wish to be. I encourage you to further explore what you can do to have the brain, and the life, you deserve and desire, and to continue the journey toward the person you are meant to be.

To Your Journey,
Alicia R. Maher, M.D.

Appendices

Understanding Treatment Options

ADHD Treatments

This book has described many ideas and strategies for improving life with ADHD and dealing with ADHD-like symptoms. In this section, I want to clearly delineate the standard treatments widely used to manage it. As I have done in the rest of the book, I will focus primarily on treatments geared toward adult ADHDers. But before jumping into treatment, let's do a quick review of some of the issues associated with diagnosis.

Properly diagnosing ADHD is difficult because of the lack of objective tests available to easily identify it. As we saw in the overview, the diagnosis of ADHD involves a particular set of symptoms and behaviors manifested over a certain period of time at a certain level of severity. What makes diagnosis tricky, as many people have experienced firsthand, is that ADHD symptoms can occur, to a lesser extent, in non-ADHDers.

When ADHD is the diagnosis, there are basically three treatment options to address the symptoms:

- Medication
- Behavior modification
- Alternative treatments (herbal supplements & diet)

The advice in this book primarily describes behavior modification techniques to manage ADHD and/or ADHD-like symptoms in non-ADHDers.

However, this section is aimed at those who have been diagnosed with ADD or ADHD by a competent professional who is trained to make such a diagnosis. Furthermore, the information here is not considered sufficient to make decisions with respect to individual treatment options. Rather, it should be used as a basis for further discussion of treatment with a prescribing physician.

In my practice, I have adopted the attitude that medication should be used only when absolutely necessary. If there is any other way of managing a disease or disorder in the mind or body, it should be tried first. That holds true for the symptoms of ADHD—to a certain extent. While research has shown that behavioral management/modification techniques, including the skills and practices suggested in this book, are important complements to medication treatment, they are not sufficient on their own to alleviate the symptoms of ADHD. To do so, they should be accompanied by medication treatment, particularly in the beginning, while the techniques are being established, practiced and integrated into an individual's daily life.

Given the high potential for significant negative consequences (e.g. increased substance abuse, relationship disruptions and divorce, higher probability of arrests and/or accidents), in individuals with ADHD who are not treated with medication, I believe it's important not to delay considering options other than behavioral modification alone. In my experience, medication is, in most cases, a must to effectively treat ADHD. That's not to say changing behaviors and learning the skills to do so aren't also important. Plus, they should still be practiced while other treatments are being utilized.

One way of conceptualizing this is my "Row, row, row your boat" analogy. Imagine two people standing on the edge of a lake. They both want to get to the other side. The non-ADHDer has a boat to row across; the ADHDer does not. Sure, the ADHDer could swim across the lake, but the water is cold, and it's going to take a heckuva' lot more effort to swim than it will to row. Giving an ADHDer medication is like giving her a boat that she can row across the lake so she doesn't have to swim. But just getting into the boat won't get the ADHDer across the lake–she has to row the boat to go anywhere. To row the boat she needs oars; she also needs to know how to use them. Furthermore, giving someone a boat, oars and the knowhow to use them won't get them across the lake, any more than giving someone a pen, paper and the ability to write will cause them to produce a novel. In addition to the boat, the oars and the knowledge to use them, the ADHDer must also be motivated to get across the lake. Giving an ADHDer behavioral skills without medication is like giving her oars without a boat.

If medication is the best way to treat ADHD, why is there resistance in many quarters to its use, particularly in treating children? It's easy to understand why some people would not want to use controlled substances as their first choice in treating an illness, especially when treating a child. I myself resisted taking prescription medication for many years, choosing instead over-the-counter stimulants and a stimulating antidepressant, until difficulties at work forced me to explore other options. But when I experienced the life improvements made possible through proper medication treatment, I wished I had taken it much sooner. I try not to think of how much easier and effective I could have been had I chosen to use medication years earlier.

As I went through life, I diligently acquired the skills in this book and struggled to put them into practice with mixed success. I would be organized for a while, but lacked the follow-through to make the strategies stick and thus create lasting habits and behavior patterns that would have served me well. Without a boat, I was flailing around in the lake with a set of oars, which sometimes helped me to float, but were essentially useless in getting me where I wanted to go. It was a REAL struggle, and to be honest, I often felt like I was drowning.

One of the most painful consequences of swimming/flailing instead of rowing is how it can damage one's self-esteem. ADHDers often try everything to make themselves function like others, and judge themselves failures when they can't "get it together." When they aren't diagnosed, ADHDers often feel lazy and incompetent and wonder if there is something inherently wrong with them.

Treatment with medication can help change that. The variety of medications used to treat ADHD fall into two groups: stimulants and non-stimulants. Research consistently shows stimulants are more effective in treating ADHD than non-stimulants. However, everyone's biological and social circumstances are unique, and it's difficult to predict how different individuals will respond to specific medications. Therefore, some "experimentation" may be needed to determine which medication at which dosage level is best for any given individual. If, given sufficient time, one medication doesn't produce the desired results, it's best to try another.

Before getting into specific options and how they work, I'd like to clarify what medication can and cannot do. The medications available to treat both ADHD adults and children are similar, and equally effective in managing symptoms. However, the level of effectiveness is sometimes more difficult to quantify in adults than in children, because there are fewer objective measures, such as school grades, by which to evaluate outcomes.

What can one expect from the treatment of adult ADHDers with medication? I laughed at a routine by comedian Mitch Hedberg based on him imagining taking ADHD medication he didn't need. He wondered if it would make him so focused that he would frustrate friends and family by begging them for more details whenever they tried to tell him a story.

Though humorous, the scenario he lampooned wouldn't occur in real life. It's true; ADHD medications may enhance the ability of non-ADHDers to concentrate and focus, and some wish to use them when they have a paper to write, a report to prepare, or an exam to pass. Additionally, some people want to take ADHD medication "for the fun of it," as a way to get "high." One of my patients told me she was asked by fellow college students to sell them her Ritalin, and had been offered as much as $20 per pill. While the medication made her focus and slowed her down (an effect she didn't like), it made her colleagues feel more stimulated and "up." It's also noteworthy that, while ADHDers can be treated effectively for decades with the same dosage, non-ADHDers become tolerant to the medication and must keep increasing the dose to get the same stimulating effect over the long term.

As the areas of the brain involved with cognition are generally more sensitive to medication than the areas tied to hyperactivity, the first effects of medication are usually noticed in attentiveness. Taking medication should result in an ability to focus more on tasks. As concentration improves, those who take medication are less distracted by what goes on around them, and are able to focus for longer. This ability, however, has limitations. An ADHDer on the proper medication may be less likely to daydream. However, in today's age of overwhelming stimulation, even non-ADHDers are more easily distracted and scattered. Plus, our brains are not designed to focus for long periods; we need breaks to maintain concentration.

Improvements in physical symptoms include better coordination and/ or less of the "klutziness" which often accompanies ADHD, as well as less difficulty sleeping at night, and an easier time getting going in the morning. Nevertheless, sleep issues are among the side effects of some medication (see below).

ADHDers on medication are also usually less impulsive, less physically hyperactive and more self-controlled. They are generally more able to think through statements and actions before making them.

Medication can also help ease the emotional symptoms associated with ADHD to a degree that can be felt by the ADHDer and observed by those around them. ADHDers often experience excessive irritability, and, as we have seen, they have a low tolerance for frustration. Together, or separately, these symptoms can lead to episodic emotional outbursts that cause interpersonal problems for ADHDers. The person taking the medication, as well as others around him or her, should notice the ADHDer is less angry, less often. There should also be a noticeable decrease in the pervasive and difficult-to-explain negativity associated with ADHD.

The effects on emotional symptoms bring me to an important point: the medication-induced changes might be less noticeable to the ADHDer than to his family, friends and colleagues. For the most part, the significant others of my ADHD patients express much more excitement and enthusiasm about the effects of treatment than my patients do! ADHDers often do not notice the changes wrought by medication. They continue to do whatever comes naturally, and fail to realize what comes naturally is quite different when they take medication than when they do not.

Besides the emotional impacts others appreciate, there's usually a noticeable decrease in verbal and behavioral impulsivity. The result is a vast improvement in conversations with the ADHDer. She will be better able to avoid interrupting others, as well as to take in what is being said. In the workplace, the ADHDer on the correct medication will experience a generally improved ability to function and complete tasks–likely due to improved concentration and focus.

ADHDers are often highly motivated to take medication to alleviate a particularly problematic symptom. However, when taking medication, one should remember that, just as several symptoms must occur together to diagnose ADHD, so should treatment resolve several symptoms. Alleviating the most problematic symptom is not sufficient to consider the illness itself has been treated. While not all symptoms may be resolved, treatment is considered successful only if it results in the individual no longer meet the criteria for a diagnosis of ADHD. If this is not the case, it usually means either a higher dose of the medication or a switch to another medication is required. It's important to restate that the ADHDer himself is not a reliable source for gauging the effectiveness of medication, as he may not feel he is behaving any differently. Input from others in a position to observe behavioral changes in the ADHDer is essential to determine the true effect (or lack thereof) of any given treatment.

That sums up what medication should do. So what does it *not* do? There's nothing magical about ADHD medication–it does not give ADHDers any mental advantages or disadvantages. It merely makes their brains more functionally similar to non-ADHDers. The purpose of taking medication is to manage symptoms, so an individual's true potential may be expressed. Once the correct dosage reduces troublesome ADHD symptoms, increasing the dosage (and thus the neurochemicals) provides no additional benefit.

Medication also does not make people smarter. ADHDers have a hard time making full use of their intellectual abilities because of the disorder. When their brain functioning is brought to its full potential with proper medication, their natural intellect becomes more obvious. In the same way, medication does not guarantee enhanced career success. However, by reducing their symptoms, ADHDers who take medication are often better able to keep up with job demands, thus making greater success more likely.

In the chapter on social skills, we saw how inattentiveness causes communication issues. ADHDers on medication should become noticeably more attentive. However, medication won't instantly make them great conversationalists or erase the years of bad communication habits. Remember also: inattentiveness is not confined to ADHDers! Many non-ADHDers also find it hard to resist constantly checking their electronic devices during conversations. The inattentiveness caused by the neurobiology of ADHD can easily be replaced by the endless distractions of modern life. Medication helps ADHDers be more attentive, but they must also practice good communication skills (i.e. they have to use good communication "oars" to row their conversational "boats.")

Now let's move on to the two main classes of medication options: stimulants and non-stimulant, of which the former have been found to be more effective overall in the treatment of ADHD.

STIMULANTS

Stimulant medications to treat ADHD are either methylphenidate or amphetamine based. If you choose to take a stimulant, determining the best one for you may require some experimentation (with the guidance of your prescribing physician). Clearly, your goal should be the best results with the fewest side effects. You will likely take the medication over the long term, so it makes sense to take your time to find the best medication for you. Don't give up too soon! Once you find the right medication, you then need to determine the right dosage. This takes time and patience.

One of the questions I am most frequently asked about stimulant medication is whether its effects wear off over time. The answer is no. ADHDers do not show tolerance to stimulants. The dose may need to be increased a few times in the beginning, but this is not due to a loss of effectiveness; it's simply a matter of finding the correct dose for the individual. As the dose is "upped," one can expect to have gradually greater effects in an increasing number of symptom areas. Once the optimal dose is discovered, it can be maintained indefinitely.

The effects of stimulant medications are felt from the first dose, but it may take several weeks to achieve maximal benefit. This delay may be partly due to neuronal modulation, as well as to the fact that while some symptoms are corrected, others become more apparent. For example, as the ADHDer becomes better able to complete tasks, the pile-up of previously uncompleted tasks may seem daunting. The medication is working, but the newly medicated ADHDer may feel overwhelmed until he gets on top of things.

Taking medication may also cause side effects related to an improvement in symptoms. For example, some of my patients say treatment with stimulants has (surprisingly to them but not to me) caused them to feel sleepy. One patient became so sedated she began taking her medication at night. How could a stimulating medication lead to sleepiness? Remember: contrary to "normal" people, ADHDers feel slowed down when they take stimulants. This patient was a dramatic example of that–the medication slowed her down to such a degree she realized how sleepy she really was. Her ADHD hyperactivity had kept her sufficiently agitated to get through each day, but she had accumulated a significant sleep deficit. Even as the medication takes effect and the individual begins to function more normally, the real and complete effect may not be evident until she comes back into balance, which can sometimes take several weeks.

METHYLPHENIDATE-BASED STIMULANTS

The first of the two stimulant types we'll cover are the methylphenidate-based stimulants; they include Ritalin, and similar medications. The main difference between the various medications in this group is how long they last. They all contain methylphenidate, but the form is different. For example, Ritalin and Methylin are both names for methylphenidate in its basic, immediate-release form. Methylphenidate is relatively short acting: in most people, it begins to work about 30 minutes after being ingested. However, when taken with food, its absorption, and therefore the onset of action, may be delayed two to three hours. That's why people often prefer to take it when they wake up, before they eat. Methylphenidate tends to have the strongest effect about two hours later, and is finally released about four hours after being taken; it thus works well for someone who only requires four hours of symptom control. If longer-term symptom relief is needed, such as for an eight-hour workday, methylphenidate must be taken again after about four hours. If symptom control is also required in the evenings, a third dose may be needed. As I've mentioned, experimentation (in consultation with the prescribing physician, of course) will help determine the optimal dosage and frequency.

Because many people find it inconvenient to take medication multiple times daily, manufacturers have developed longer-acting forms of methylphenidate-type medications. They pills still contain methylphenidate, but are made so the medication is delivered over a longer period. For example, time-released Concerta partially dissolves, and starts to have an effect about 30 minutes after it's taken. The rest of the methylphenidate is "pushed" out as an inner "compartment" of the tablet fills with gastric juice over the course of the day; the effect is much like taking a second and third pill.

These longer-acting versions of methylphenidate medications are classified based on whether they are extended release (eight-hour effects) or sustained release (12-hour effects). The extended-release medications include Ritalin SR, Methylin ER, and Metadate ER; the sustained-release type includes Concerta, Ritalin LA, and Metadate CD.

Methylphenidate may also be delivered in a patch form known as Daytrana, which delivers the medication through the skin. It's most often used in children, and usually applied to the hip. Because the medication is absorbed through the skin, it may lead to fewer gastrointestinal side effects (see below). However, it may also take longer to act, and should be applied two hours prior to when its effect is required. Daytrana symptom relief can last around nine hours. As the most extensive testing of this type of medication has been done in children, you should work closely with your prescribing physician to determine if it is right for you.

Finally, the methylphenidate molecule itself can be altered to produce the same effects with less medication. In addition to immediate-release, Focalin is available in a longer-acting version called Focalin XR.

AMPHETAMINE-BASED STIMULANTS

The other type of stimulant medication is amphetamine based. Different forms of the amphetamine molecule produce the various medications in this class. The most commonly referred from this group is Adderall, the generic name of which is dextroamphetamine/amphetamine. The regular form of Adderall lasts for three to six hours, while an extended form, Adderal XR, lasts for up to eight. Other forms, called dextroamphetamine, comprise just part of the amphetamine molecule; they include Dexedrine and Dextrostat, as well as the longer-acting Dexodrine SR and Dexedrine Spansule. It is also available in liquid form (e.g. Procentra), for those who have trouble swallowing tablets, as well as in a form that requires digestion to be active (e.g. Vyvanse). Vyvanse was developed to prevent the potential misuse of ADHD medication by non-ADHDers. As ADHD medications can potentially be misused by crushing them, and either snorting or injecting them to get a "high," medication manufacturers research ways to avert misuse. Vyvanse is a "prodrug" that requires digestion to be active. This means it can only be used in the slower-acting oral form, making it difficult to achieve a "high" from taking it.

Although ADHD *brains* process the stimulating neurochemicals differently (thus making ADHDers on medication calmer rather than more stimulated), ADHDer *bodies* process them the same way as non-ADHDer bodies. Therefore, though the mind is slower and calmer, the body may be stimulated, leading to an increased heart rate and other symptoms of stimulation. Though these side effects are common, not everyone experiences them; they tend to occur at the beginning of treatment, and become less noticeable over time. Although no tolerance to the mental effects of these medications should develop, tolerance to the physical side effects may occur (e.g. loss of appetite might be an immediate side effect that could subside over time).

The physical side effects of include nervousness, irritability, general overstimulation, restlessness, difficulty sleeping, and tremor or shakiness of the hands, as well as headache, dizziness, abdominal pain, nausea, weight loss, blurred vision, dry mouth, and even seizures. In people who already have vocal or motor tics, such as those with Tourette's syndrome, taking a stimulant can make those tics worse. In very rare cases, stimulants may cause suicidal thinking. Even more rare still, stimulants may cause someone to have mania or an emergency situation called neuroleptic malignant syndrome, where the muscles stiffen and can't relax. Particularly in those with preexisting issues of the heart, there can be serious cardiac side effects, even sudden death. That's why it's *critical* for anyone with a suspected heart condition to have a cardiac evaluation prior to taking any kind of stimulant.

The number of possible side effects extends past what I cover in this book. Generally, if you feel something unusual happening within the first couple of weeks of taking ADHD medication, you should talk about it with your prescribing physician to determine whether it is a side effect. If the stimulant then needs to be discontinued, it is best to slowly taper down the dose instead of abruptly stopping it to avoid withdrawal effects.

MANAGING SIDE EFFECTS

So how might one manage the most commonly occurring side effects? Besides switching medications, there are several ways to do so.

As these medications were initially developed as appetite suppressants, decreased appetite is a common side effect. This has been more of an issue in children, as few adults seem to mind a decline in appetite. However, if this is an issue for you, eating prior to taking the medication is one way to avert loss of appetite.

Irritability is another side effect, particularly with shorter acting stimulants. It primarily occurs as the stimulant level drops prior to taking the next dose. As the medication goes out of the system, a slight withdrawal effect occurs, leading to irritability. One remedy is to switch to a longer-acting stimulant, which is released over a longer period and leaves the system more gradually, thus causing smaller variations in medication levels and therefore less irritability.

Some people also suffer insomnia. If you have difficulty falling asleep at night, you might want to try a shorter-acting medication and take your last dose no less than six hours before your intended bedtime. This allows the medication to be metabolized out of your system before you are ready to sleep.

For effects such as tremulousness/shaking, some people take a "beta-blocker." However, this is a cardiac medication that should, like all medications, only be taken under a physician's guidance, and after potential cardiac issues have been addressed.

NON-STIMULANTS

In general, non-stimulant medications have not been found to be as effective, overall, as stimulants. However, there are a variety of reasons that some ADHDers may choose non-stimulants over stimulants.

The availability of stimulants is strictly regulated because of the potential abuse issues. In the United States, restricted access means prescriptions for stimulants cannot be called into a pharmacy, nor can they be refilled. As a result, individuals taking stimulant medication must schedule and attend regular appointments and keep track of a paper script, which must be presented at the pharmacy in person. They can't get more than one month's supply of medication at a time, which means they won't have any extra medication on hand in case some is lost. They also can't fill their prescriptions in advance to stockpile a supply in the event of extended travel to destinations where it might be difficult to get prescriptions filled.

All of these issues can be difficult for a newly diagnosed ADHDer who may have trouble keeping track of the details of life before his or her symptoms are managed with the help of medication (a bit of a catch-22 as it were!).

Even those who have been on medication for decades may find these issues to be too much of a hassle. For these reasons, some people may prefer to take a non-stimulant, which may be more effective and have certain advantages for particular individuals.

For adults, the main types of non-stimulant medication include modafinil, atomoxetine, antidepressant medications that have stimulating properties, and adrenergic agonists, although the latter are primarily used in hyperactive children. There are quite a few other types of medications, too many to cover individually here, so I will confine the discussion to those most commonly used.

Modafinil is a stimulant-like non-stimulant; it comes in different forms under the brand names Provigil and Nuvigil.

Atomoxetine, or Strattera, allows more of the neurochemicals needed in the higher-ordered thinking part of the brain without increasing them in the "feel-good" part of the brain. Because it doesn't lead to a high and doesn't have the abuse potential stimulants do, it is not classified as such. Unlike stimulants, which act immediately, atomoxetine takes several weeks to have an effect. Not knowing this, many people give up on this medication too quickly, before it's had a chance to work.

Though much weaker than stimulants, some antidepressant medications also act to increase the stimulating neurochemicals and may have some effect on the symptoms of ADHD. These include bupropion (best known as Wellbutrin), venlafaxine (Effexor), and duloxetine (Cymbalta), as well as desipramine, nortriptyline, and imipramine.

Finally, the adrenergic agonists, such as clonidine and guanfacine (or Intuniv), can enhance stimulating neurochemicals, but are mostly used in children rather than adults.

Like stimulants, non-stimulants have side effects, which should be discussed with one's physician before starting treatment.

To close this section on medication, it's worth mentioning that not everyone who has ADHD wants to be treated for its symptoms. Some ADHDers try treatment and decide not to continue it, with the knowledge they could be "like everyone else" if they chose to be. I know one man in particular whose business it is to be zany and off the cuff, even inappropriate at times; his chosen profession rewards for his impulsivity. He has decided (at least for now) not to take medication (much to the disappointment of his long-suffering wife) to be at his best in his career. When those around him wonder "what's wrong" with him, he responds to their comments with good-natured humor, knowing he has made a conscious choice to be as he is. Still, trying medication was a boon: after years of questioning himself for his poor academic performance, he finally discovered the cause. He also knew he could treat it if he wanted. The knowledge was a huge boost to his self-esteem. As long as he knows he can be "normal," he feels as capable as anyone else.

BEHAVIORAL TREATMENTS

We've covered many of the behavioral treatments for ADHD and ADHD-like symptoms in the core of the book. They are designed to provide structure and teach skills to help ADHDers and non-ADHDers with ADHD-like symptoms better manage their lives. By increasing awareness of ineffective habits and teaching organizational and other skills, behavioral treatments are of paramount importance in the treatment of ADHD. That said, they have not been consistently validated as effective treatments of ADHD when used alone. As we saw in the "Row, row, row your boat" analogy, using behavioral skills without medication is like giving someone oars and teaching her to row, then putting her on the shoreline without a boat and asking her to get to the other side. Behavior modification can certainly improve an ADHDer's life, but it's probably not enough on its own, and should be used in conjunction with other treatments, such as medication therapy.

Often, it is difficult for ADHDers to effectively implement behavioral skills until they are stabilized by medication. However, the more an ADHDer is able to discover ways to organize himself, schedule tasks, make lists, keep a calendar, manage time, etc., the better off he will be and the less medication he may require. This is particularly true of ADHDers who were not diagnosed as children, or who did not start receiving treatment until adulthood.

Besides using a book such as this to become aware of and learn new skills, ADHDers who wish to make these kinds of lifestyle changes may choose counseling, psychotherapy, and/or working with a life coach specializing in ADHD. Professionals in these areas help ADHDers create and implement goals to change and improve their lives. They work closely with ADHD clients, provide structure, facilitate learning, teach skills and "cheerlead" as needed.

ALTERNATIVE TREATMENTS

Herbal Supplements

In addition to medication and behavior management, alternative treatments (the efficacy of which remains unproven) also exist. In the interest of thoroughness, I want to discuss some of them.

Besides meditation, yoga and other practices designed to center and calm the self, certain herbal supplements have been proposed to treat ADHD. I have not found compelling research placing their effectiveness at the same level as medication, and I want to be clear I am not recommending them as an alternative to medication. You may wish to consider them if you have noticed symptoms consistent with ADHD, but you do not meet the full diagnosis—perhaps you just want a boost in concentration, but aren't at risk of losing your job or marriage because of your ADHD-like behavior.

Anyone who considers taking medication and/or herbal supplements of any kind should do so with caution. In the case of the latter, I recommend being especially vigilant and aware of potential safety issues. Know that just because something is described as "natural" does not necessarily mean that it is safe. For example, in 2004, the Food and Drug Administration banned the use of the natural stimulant ephedra when it was believed to have caused deaths by stroke. Research into the ingredients of herbal supplements has found ones containing unlisted ingredients, including ephedra, as well as pharmaceutical agents and other contaminants. Likewise, there are reports of supplements not containing the amount of active ingredient listed on the packaging. In treating any condition the symptoms of which are severe enough to require treatment, those ingesting a substance to treat it must ensure they take the correct dosage. Therefore, one should be cautious with products the contents of which may vary from one batch to the next.

Keeping those issues in mind, let's look at some of the proposed alternatives. For the most part, they are stimulating herbs, the effect of which is milder than amphetamine-based stimulants, which must be prescribed. They include cola nut (Cola nitida), country mallow, pinellia, and seville (bitter orange). Caffeine also acts as a mild stimulant and can affect concentration (there are many well-known caffeine-containing beverages or over-the-counter preparations to boost your energy and keep you awake). Some herbs also contain caffeine; they include guarana (Paullinia cupana), yerba mate (Ilex papguariensis), and again, cola nut.

Another proposed supplement is zinc, which research has shown to have some effect in children who take it with other ADHD treatment. It seems to reduce hyperactivity and impulsivity symptoms more than those of inattention. Zinc can be taken as a supplement or consumed through the diet in red meat, poultry, seafood, dairy products, beans, nuts, and whole grains.

Fish oil, which contains omega-3 fatty acids, provides a variety of benefits to many areas of the body, and has also been suggested as an aid to addressing ADHD symptoms. Ongoing research is looking into the effects of fatty acids in various psychiatric conditions, as they seem to have a stabilizing effect on the coverings of the neurons, or brain cells. This stabilizing effect may help with neuronal function and, theoretically, provide a benefit to ADHDers. More research needs to be done, but this is an area to watch, and, given all of the possible physical benefits of omega-3s, I am apt to encourage anyone to take it for overall good health.

Supplements for conditions associated with ADHD (e.g. sleeplessness), include substances such as melatonin, which may help some people sleep, and thus improve concentration and mood, and decrease restlessness. If sleep improvements alone are sufficient to address an individual's symptoms, they were unlikely to have been caused by ADHD. Nevertheless, anything that can be done to alleviate ADHD and ADHD-like symptoms is obviously beneficial.

One supplement research has shown to have no benefit is St John's wort, though it is used to treat other mental health conditions due to its effect on neurochemistry.

Diet

Whether or not supplements are effective in treating ADHD is questionable; the same is true of diet. For decades, people have speculated that some foods (i.e. those containing preservatives or food coloring; or those high in simple sugars) may exacerbate ADHD. However, several controlled studies have found no adequate data to confirm this theory.

Nevertheless, many people believe (erroneously) that sugar causes hyperactivity. This may be because many children are more active (even hyperactive) when they eat sugary foods. Though decreasing sugar intake may make children less agitated, it does not cure the ADHD symptoms. If reducing sugar alone stops the ADHD-like symptoms in a child, I would question the diagnosis. The hyperactive behaviors may look the same, but the cause is completely different: in ADHD it is the brain's altered way of processing of neurochemicals. I would expect the effects of altered neurochemical processing (i.e. hyperactivity) to remain, even if sugar is completely eliminated in the diet of a child with ADHD.

Processed foods have also been implicated as a potential cause of ADHD. This may be because they tend to cause energy swings due to the way they are digested. As they contain little fiber, processed foods are easily broken down once eaten and often cause an immediate insulin and energy surge, which can look like hyperactivity. Likewise, the way they are rapidly digested leads to a "crash" following the "high." This sudden decrease in energy may look like inattention. Though eliminating these foods won't cure ADHD, it may help manage symptoms they exacerbate.

Some people also suggest limiting the ingestion of foods containing glutamate helps alleviate the symptoms of ADHD. The neurochemical glutamate is known to be activating in the brain, and at normal levels allows the brain to function effectively. The proposed theory is too much glutamate causes too much brain activation. Though this wouldn't cause ADHD, it could possibly augment the symptoms. This is an interesting area to explore; however, at this time, there is insufficient evidence to recommend it.

Useful Excercises

1. Use Technology as a Motivator
2. Unplug
3. Create "To Do" Lists & Calendars (& Delegate When Possible!)
4. Put Things in Their Place
5. Schedule & Manage Your Time
6. Create Affirmations
7. Communicate by Mirroring More
8. Beware of Cognitive Distortions
9. "Upscale" Your Thoughts
10. Breathe into Relaxation with Pranayama
11. Use Mindfulness to Be More Aware
12. Relax Each & Every Part of You
13. List Your Great Ideas
14. Do What Works
15. Define & Work Towards Goals

1. Use Technology as a Motivator

What is irresistible to *you*? What do you look forward to and enjoy immensely? We've focused on technology, but, so long as it doesn't lead to obesity, lung cancer, or rehab, feel free to choose anything else that can be done throughout the day to keep you motivated. If you don't know where to start, try the examples described here. Turn your phone off or set it so that you won't hear whether or not you are receiving texts or voicemails or e-mails, or alerts from your social networking applications and/or sites. Or, make it so that you can't see whether or not you are receiving e-mail on your computer.

Make a commitment to yourself to do a certain amount of a necessary task before checking your phone, computer, or networking site. Be sure to have a limit if you're using the social networking site as a reward, such as only checking messages or reading only one page of updates, so that you don't end up distracted off of your original task.

Take Action

Choose something that currently gets you distracted to use as a motivator, such as one of the examples above. Write how you will use this to motivate you, such as checking only after a certain task is completed:

_____

_____

_____

Notice if this had any positive effects and write them here. The act of writing them acknowledges them on a deeper level, which can assist in motivating you to continue the practice:

_____

_____

_____

Mark here when you have completed 30 days of arranging a motivator around one task each day.

_____ Thirty Days Completed

Congratulations!

2. UNPLUG

Part of effective time management is knowing when to do an activity. It's important to determine when your brain is most effective for particular tasks. During the time that you are best able to do intellectual tasks, unplug the phone or computer, and block out other distractions.

Rather than allowing yourself to be distracted randomly throughout the day, save checking e-mails for particular times and making calls for another. After any initial fears of missing something important wear off, many people feel a greater sense of control over their lives, knowing that they can only be bothered at particular times. This should also help to increase your sense of focus and complete tasks more readily.

Take Action

List activities that you need to complete each day. Make a second list of distractions and how you will control them (i.e., e-mails—check only before work, during lunch, and once in the evening).

Activities to complete

_____

_____

_____

Distractions and how to control

_____

_____

_____

Mark when you have completed 30 days in a row of controlling one distraction.

_____ Thirty Days Completed

Bravo—you did it!

3. CREATE "TO DO" LISTS & CALENDARS (AND DELEGATE WHEN POSSIBLE!)

List making is an essential component of organization. Lists are particularly helpful for decreasing forgetfulness and increasing the likelihood of follow-through. When it is difficult to keep track of details, lists take the thinking out of remembering. By making a to-do list each day, you can see how much needs to be done and allot adequate time to do it.

One way of enhancing a to-do list even further is by dividing up items into what *must* be done and what it would be *nice to do*, or what needs to be done at work versus what needs to be done at home, or even what is enjoyable versus what is draining. By having lists, you never need to worry that you will forget to do something.

Lists can also help you get organized. For example, making a list of work projects will make sure that anything that is needed will get done. A grocery list ensures needed items can be written down, so they will be remembered on shopping day. You can also start lists for holidays or travel items–write things down as they occur to you so you are less stressed trying to remember things at the last minute.

Create your lists in a way that ensures you will look at them. A notepad on the fridge, a notebook you carry with you, the notes function available on most phones or computers, all work well as long as they are with you when you think of the things you must remember. You may choose to use a combination of strategies for different purposes (e.g. a grocery list on the fridge, an overall to do list on your phone).

If, when you review your lists, you find the number of tasks daunting, it's time to delegate. Ask yourself if there are tasks that could be done as well if not better by someone else. Could the housework be done by a cleaning service? Might your partner pick up the dry cleaning on the way home from work every second Tuesday? Could a team member at work do part of the research needed for an ongoing project? If yes, get those tasks off your lists and onto theirs! Equally, you may also find items on your list that others have delegated to you. Make sure you don't accept tasks if you don't have time to do them: in other words, learn to say no. The objective of delegation is to end up with the tasks that are most suited to our abilities. If you try to do it all, you'll be less effective.

Keep a calendar too. Record in advance what you must remember so you to have all the necessary information when and where you need it on the day. For example, on the date of an event put the event address and location, the venue phone number, what you need to bring, the dress code, etc., to avoid the stress of having to recall it all on the day.

Take Action

Make at least one list each day (e.g. a to-do list, a grocery list), or be more detailed in the calendar that you keep; update your list daily. The more that you practice using a list, the more you will discover ways to make lists work for you. Consistency is the key to success.

Write one area where you will keep a daily list:

_____

_____

_____

Decide the best place to keep your list (e.g. on paper, electronically):

_____

After you've completed 30 days, mark it here. Then, think of other lists that would be helpful and list them.

_____ Thirty Days Completed

Yes! You are a superstar.

Additional lists that would be helpful:

_____

_____

_____

4. PUT THINGS IN THEIR PLACE

Organizing your belongings will make life easier and less stressful. Imagine eliminating the frustrating experience of not being able to find your keys. Or, think of how much less stressful packing would be if you knew you always had what you needed.

I like the saying "A place for everything, and everything in its place." Having a particular place for everything and returning it to that place when you are done using it means you never have to wonder where it is. Always keep frequently used items such as keys, in the same easy-to-access (a hook by the door for example). If several things are needed each time you go out, have an organizing center (or even just a shelf) by the door. Items placed there will be easily available when you come and go.

Likewise, keeping all the items required for one activity together in one place ensures they're readily available when you need them. For example, if you enjoy skiing, have a box or bag with all your skiing gear–you won't have to search high and low for all your ski stuff the next time you hit the slopes. Having everything you need to pay bills available in one box can also stream-line the process when you sit down to deal with your account. Even keeping items in a particular place in your car or purse means always knowing where they are–so long as you return them, of course!

Take Action

List items that you often search for, along with a place where each item can be kept:

_____

_____

_____

List an activity, frequent trip, or place you go that requires you to remember several items. Then write an idea for a way to house all of the needed items together (a box, bag, particular drawer, etc.):

_____

_____

_____

As organizational ideas are widely available, list others here that you know would be helpful, but haven't committed to trying (yet!):

_____

_____

_____

Now, commit to 30 days of: returning an item to a particular place each day, keeping a designated place for items related to an activity, or another organizational idea. The important thing is to commit to daily use of the technique. List what you will commit to doing, and mark when 30 days in a row have been completed:

_____

_____

_____

_____ Thirty Days Completed

I bet you feel more organized already!

5. SCHEDULE & MANAGE YOUR TIME

Choosing the best time to complete tasks is a big factor in whether or not (and how well), things get done. ADHDer or not, there are times during the day when the neurochemical milieu of your brain is more conducive to doing certain tasks rather than others.

There are two key components to time management: knowing what needs to be done, and determining when to do it. Generally, we tend to figure out what needs to be done and how long each item will take, and then we start going about doing those items. If, however, we also think about the best time to do each item, we can complete them more efficiently, using less energy. If you are most able to concentrate in the morning, it may be best to save tasks requiring concentration to the following day, rather than struggling to complete them in the afternoon or evening. If a task is pleasant, it might be best to do that task at a time when your energy is lowest, when you are less able to do other tasks.

Take Action

List tasks you must do during a typical day. For example, returning calls/ e-mails, particular tasks at work, home-related tasks, paying bills, etc.:

_____

_____

_____

Using the list above, group the tasks according to when it is best for you to complete them.

Morning tasks:

_____

_____

_____

During-work tasks

_____

_____

_____

Right-after-work tasks

_____

_____

_____

Evening tasks

_____

_____

_____

Arrange your tasks daily for 30 days. It might take several tries before you know when the best time is for a particular task. Not to worry; what is important is developing an awareness of your own ideal schedule and then consistently applying it.

_____ Thirty Days Completed

Well done!

6. Create Affirmations

If your way of being with others doesn't seem to work for you and you want to change, it is helpful to affirm the way you desire to be. Often, when people decide something needs to be changed about themselves, they start by focusing on what is "wrong." This is less effective and less motivating than focusing on the positives.

Affirmations are powerful change-makers. Why? Because the brain does not know whether we are *actually* experiencing something or just *thinking* about experiencing it. That's why athletes "practice" a routine in their minds before they actually perform it. Visualizing a great outcome helps increase their chance of achieving it. In the same way, making an affirmation of the way you want to be helps you to experience that way of being in your mind and increases your chances of actually becoming that way.

Not using this powerful ability of our minds to change our lives is akin to taking a long journey by car and only using first gear. We may eventually reach our destination, but the drive will be slow and inefficient. To engage all the gears in your life journey and experience a different way of being, utilize your brain's ability to imagine yourself acting from your desired state of being.

Once you know the way you would like to be, create a statement describing it. One of the most famous affirmation statements is "every day, in every way, I'm getting better." Make sure that the statement is in the present tense and positive—i.e., affirming what you do want, rather than saying what you don't want. Repeat it aloud several times a day, every day, forever!

Take Action

Take a few minutes to do a meditation. Close your eyes and imagine yourself acting from the way you want to be. This may be happier, calmer, or any other way you choose. Make sure you draw in as many senses as possible to get into your desired state. Imagine how things would look, sound, smell, and feel. Write a description of your desired state here:

_____

_____

_____

Create an affirmation statement that captures your desired state. Make sure it is in the present tense and states what you do want, rather than what you don't want (e.g. "I feel confident and comfortable making presentations,"

NOT "I don't want to feel afraid of public speaking"). Write your statement here:

_____

_____

_____

Commit to stating your affirmation several times per day.

It helps to write the statement down on cards and place them in the bathroom, on the refrigerator, and in other places where you will see and read the statement often.

Mark here after you have said your affirmation at least once daily for 30 days.

_____ Thirty Days Completed

Congratulations on getting better every day!

7. COMMUNICATE MORE EFFECTIVELY BY MIRRORING

Good communication skills do not necessarily come naturally for anyone, but can be particularly difficult for those who have had to deal with impulsivity and attention deficit in their formative years. Much has been written on this topic, and many resources are available; here are a few ideas to get you started:

It is important to listen when someone else speaks. Looking at this from the perspective of social skills, it is equally important that the speaker feels listened to. Using mirroring is one way of making speakers feel heard. Mirroring can be done both nonverbally and verbally.

Nonverbal mirroring involves imitating the facial expressions, posture, and mannerisms of the speaker. Try also to match their tone of voice, volume, and speed. The goal is to feel others' experiences. (Hint: don't get so involved in trying to imitate that you let yourself get distracted from what is being said.)

Verbal monitoring is also useful. Listen to the words the speaker uses and incorporate some of them into your answers. Listening to the words uses a different part of the brain than the part that creates a response. Often, while someone speaks, we engage the part of the brain that analyzes and creates a response; this prevents effective listening. By listening for the words to mirror, we hear what is being said before we develop our response. This improves listening, makes others feel heard, and leads to more effective communications with others.

Take Action

Practice mirroring. This may be most effective with a friend or someone else whom you trust to give you good feedback, but you can also practice on strangers, or even using the TV. Write the situations you attempted, along with how effective they seemed, here:

_____

_____

_____

After you've gained comfort with mirroring verbally and nonverbally, commit to doing it at least once daily for 30 days to hardwire it into your brain and create a natural way of being. Write examples of what you did, and when you've completed 30 days.

_____

_____

_____

_____ Thirty Days Completed

Mirror, mirror on the wall, YOU have become the greatest listener of all!

8. Beware of Cognitive Distortions

These top 10 "distorted" ways of thinking lead people to react to life's circumstances with negative feelings. In case you think you don't think like this, think again! We all use cognitive distortions from time to time. Problems arise when we use them to the point that our distorted view of reality makes us unhappy. Ask yourself which of the distortions listed below you have used. The more aware you are that a thought is a distortion, the more you realize you can choose a different thought—one that might make you feel better. (Adapted from Feeling Good, by David Burns, MD (New York: Avon Books, 1999, an excellent and user-friendly resource for understanding and applying cognitive therapy techniques.)

Overgeneralization: You see a single negative event as a never-ending pattern of defeat. If a bird craps on your window, you think birds are always crapping on your window, ignoring the many days they haven't.

Disqualifying the positive: You reject positive experiences by insisting they "don't count" for some reason or other. Someone giving you a compliment is "just being nice." This allows you to maintain a negative belief even if it is contradicted.

All-or-nothing thinking: You see things in black-or-white categories. For example, if your performance falls short of perfect, you see yourself as a total failure.

Mental filter: You pick out a single negative detail and dwell on it exclusively so that your vision of all reality becomes darkened, like the drop of ink that discolors an entire cup of water.

Jumping to conclusions: You make a negative interpretation even though there are no definite facts that convincingly support your conclusion. This is done through "mind reading" (assuming the motivation behind someone's actions) and "fortune telling" (assuming a negative outcome for an event).

"Catastrophizing:" You exaggerate the importance of things (such as your goof-up or someone else's achievement), or you inappropriately shrink things until they appear tiny (your own desirable qualities or another's imperfections). This is also called "the binocular trick."

Emotional reasoning: You assume your negative emotions necessarily reflect the way things really are: "I feel it, therefore it must be true." Example: Assuming you're fat because you feel fat that day.

"Should" statements: You try to motivate yourself with "should" and "shouldn't," as if you had to be whipped and punished before you could be expected to do anything. "Musts" and "oughts" are also offenders. Example: I should exercise more; I shouldn't have eaten that piece of cake.

Labeling: Instead of describing an error, you attach a label—"I'm a loser," "she's a jerk."

Personalization: You assume yourself to be responsible for an outside event. You confuse influence with control (my child got an F because I am a terrible mother).

Take Action

Train your brain to analyze your thoughts before they lead to emotional reactions. Take a few minutes to think about a difficulty you are having in life and see what cognitive distortions you can identify in your thoughts. Write a few of them here:

_____

_____

Each day, make a point of noticing when you are using these cognitive distortions. List here what effects each statement has on your mood and how you reacted after the thought.

Situation:

_____

_____

_____

Cognitive distortion:

_____

_____

_____

How the thought made me feel:

_____

_____

_____

How I reacted:

_____

_____

_____

How I would like to have reacted:

_____

_____

_____

What thought I would need to have to lead to the more positive reaction:

_____

_____

_____

9. "Upscale" Your Thoughts

In the last activity, you analyzed your thoughts to see how they lead to reactions and affect your mood. Observing the connection between thoughts and moods is helpful. You may find yourself already automatically substituting unhelpful thoughts for other more positive ones.

One way to change your thoughts (and stabilize your mood) is to transform them using the "thought transformation scale." (See picture below.)

Make a scale of your thoughts from 1 to 10, with one being the kind of thought that causes you to feel distress and 10 being the kind of thought that, if you believed it, would make you feel serene. For example, if looking at your to do list makes you feel overwhelmed, the thought behind the feeling might be "I'll never get this done," which leads you to feel distressed. The thought "I'll never get this done" would go on the scale under the number one. A serene, level 10 thought might be "Everything will be accomplished easily and quickly."

I can almost hear your protest: "If only it were as simple as telling myself to think the level 10 thought and to feel better!" True, it's not that simple. Looking on the bright side does not immediately change your reality. It may work in the long term however—especially if you believe it! Luckily, you don't have to go from your level one to level 10 thought to feel better right away, here and now. You only have to shift your brain to think in that direction. As long as you move away from the problematic thought, towards one that is more positive, you will feel better. You want to think of the level 10 thought to know what thought you want to move towards. However, you only need to think a thought one or two levels above the one you think now to feel somewhat better. A slight shift in thought is more likely to be believable, and therefore more effective in changing your mood.

Take Action

Identify a thought that causes you to feel negatively. This could be one of the cognitive distortions you identified above.

Problem thought:

_____

_____

_____

Assign a number between 1 (causing distress) and 10 (leading to serenity) to the thought: _____

Identify a possible level 10 thought related to the situation:

_____

_____

_____

Transform your problem thought to one that is closer to the level 10 thought. The new thought doesn't need to be a 10, it just needs to be believable to make you feel somewhat better

_____

_____

_____

Repeat the more positive thought several times per day, particularly whenever the problem thought arises.

_____ Thirty Days Completed

Bravo! You're on the road to better ways of thinking!

10. Relaxation with Pranayama

This breathing exercise is based on one of the ancient yogic practices of pranayama. "Prana" is Sanskrit for life force, and "yama" refers to action. So, it is an action of the life force, pranayama draws the life force in and engages it. There are many different types of pranayama exercises; my favorite is alternate nostril breathing, which focuses on the breath while balancing breathing between the two nostrils.

The hands are held in what is called a "mudra." The idea of a mudra is to lock in the sensation or benefits of a practice. The theory is, with time, you can capture the benefits so well within the mudra that, eventually, placing the hands in the mudra alone will give the benefits of the practice. The mudra for alternate nostril breathing is to fold the first two fingers of the right hand downwards toward the palm. The interesting thing about this position is that the fingers are touching at what is called the "lung point" in Chinese medicine.

- The left hand is held with the tip of the thumb and first finger pressed together and resting on the knee. Close your eyes and get ready to relax.
- Using the thumb of the right hand, press the right nostril closed and take a deep breath in through the left nostril. This is usually done to a count of four (see the first photo on next page).
- After counting to four, close both nostrils by bringing the pinky and ring finger of the right hand to press against the left nostril. Hold your breath in this position for a count of sixteen (see the middle photo on next page).
- At the end of sixteen seconds, release the thumb from the right nostril and breathe out to a count of eight seconds (see the last photo on next page).
- Continue to do this process by then leaving the thumb off of the right nostril so that it can breathe in.
- Hold both nostrils again and then release the left nostril to breathe out.
- Breathe in through the left nostril, hold, and breathe out through the right.
- Breathe in through the right nostril, hold, and breathe out through the left.
- Continue to do this for nine rounds.

Doing the four-sixteen-eight count may be hard at first, so I suggest start with two-eight-four; the proportions are the same, and you will incur a similar benefit. Practice once daily.

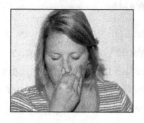 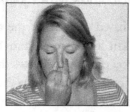 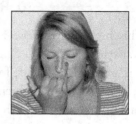

Take Action

Choose a time each day when you feel the greatest need to relax. It could be when you drive, before work, after work, even during work! Record it here. The time I most need, and can reliably complete, a session of this breathing exercise is: _____

Things that may possibly get in the way of doing this exercise daily:

_____

_____

_____

How I will manage these:

_____

_____

_____

Place a check mark here when you've done this practice once per day for 30 days in a row (don't worry if you miss a day and have to start over; just keep looking at what is getting in the way and continue until you achieve 30 consecutive days).

_____ Thirty Days Completed

Take a deep breath of congratulations!

11. USE MINDFULNESS TO BE MORE AWARE

This mindfulness practice involves eating. I like to use a raisin to demonstrate this, but other foods work equally well. The objective is to engage each of your senses in order to fully experience a particular activity. Start by looking at the raisin closely. Spend at least one minute looking at it like you've never seen one before. Notice the way the light hits it, the various grooves, any variation in color.

Next, engage your sense of smell. Hold it up to your nose and notice if there is a smell that you might not have been aware of previously.

Now, use the sense of touch. Spend another minute moving the raisin around in your fingers. Notice the consistency as you squeeze it slightly and run your fingers over the grooves.

Then, put the raisin in your mouth and feel those same grooves with the tongue, moving it around in the mouth for a while to really feel it before starting to chew. When you're ready to take a bite, notice the taste difference between how it tasted before and after biting into it. Notice as much as possible about the taste of the raisin; think of words to describe it. Savor the taste for as long as you can before you swallow it.

Now, incorporate such mindfulness into all areas of your life—notice when you are out of the present moment and engage your senses to get back into it. As you practice, you will become more adept at recognizing when you are out of your deep, still center. Do this daily, regardless of what is going on in your life. You will eventually realize there is a part of you, underneath everything else, that is unaffected by the turbulence of daily life, and you will experience life from a place of greater equanimity.

Take Action

Describe your experience of doing this exercise so that you will remember its benefits and be motivated to do it again:

_____

_____

_____

List an experience that you could use for five minutes each day to engage your senses fully. For example, you could use the eating exercise described above, or simply choose moments to observe and experience the environment around and within you.

_____

_____

_____

Place a mark here when you have completed 30 days in a row of doing five minutes of mindfulness each day.

_____ Thirty Days Completed

Kudos on being more mindful.

12. RELAX EACH AND EVERY PART OF YOU

The first step towards relaxation is to feel the difference between relaxation and tension. This exercise helps you do it. You may want to read through the exercise a few times until you can follow it without looking; alternatively, have someone read it to you. Start by slowly taking a few deep breaths in through the nose and imagine the breath filling first the abdomen and then each part of the body. Do this until you start to feel any tension fade. If it helps, give the breath a color, like golden yellow, and then imagine filling each part of your body with the color. Picturing the body helps to engage parts of your brain not involved with thinking, and gives your thinking mind a break. When you are ready, slowly tense and release each part of your body, starting with your toes and going all of the way up to each part of your face. By tensing and then releasing each part, one at a time, you feel the difference between tension and relaxation as the muscles release. Continue to do this until all of the muscles in your body have been tensed and released.

Continue to breathe and enjoy the relaxation for as long as you want, or allow yourself to drift off into sleep. When you are ready to come out of this relaxed state, slowly wiggle your fingers and toes and then roll your arms and legs, feeling energy returning to each part of your body before getting up slowly.

Remember how this relaxation feels and bring yourself back to it whenever you feel tension rising in your body.

Take Action
Describe how this relaxation exercise made you feel. Unhelpful thought: (Example: I don't want to go to work)

_____

_____

Choose a time each day when you can set aside at least five minutes to do this exercise. Just before sleep might be a good choice._____

After you have done this exercise for five minutes for 30 days in a row, make a mark here.

_____ Thirty Days Completed

Bravo!

Describe any benefits you noticed over the 30 days. This will make you more likely to make the practice a lifetime habit.

_____

_____

13. LIST YOUR GREAT IDEAS

One way to decrease the temptation to go off track when an idea occurs to you is to make a "Great Ideas" list. When an opportunity arises or an idea comes to you, it can be hard to not act on it right away. This may be due to impulsivity, the fear of forgetting it, or a general fear that you'll miss out if you don't jump on things immediately. To stop getting sidetracked, commit to completing one task before taking on any other.

Because it may be difficult to overcome the habit of switching between tasks, start by completing one task each day. Perhaps you've decided to read some articles for work, for example. Do that task without doing anything else until you're done. If something else that needs to be done occurs to you, write it down. When the one task is complete, notice if you still feel the need to do the others on your list. If not, don't do them; if so, try doing them one at a time as well.

Take Action

Choose one task and do it without allowing yourself to be sidetracked until it is complete:

_____

_____

Keep a list of other ideas that occur to you, and put them off until your task is done.

What did you notice from doing a task this way?

_____

_____

Mark here when you've completed one task without being sidetracked each day for 30 days.

_____ Thirty Days Completed!

I bet you have a great list of great ideas. . .

14. Do What Works

One of the most difficult aspects of impulsivity is the frustration of not be-ing able to do or get what you want. It's easier to tolerate, and even dissipate the frustration if you shift your focus from the experiencing the impulses to engaging the intellectual part of the brain by evaluating the situation from a different angle. One way to do this is to examine your thoughts from the per-spective of "doing what works." This isn't denying what you desire, but rather incorporating additional information about your goal into your thoughts. Retrain your brain by evaluating one frustration in this way each day for 30 days using the following exercise.

Take Action

Identify one frustration you currently experience that you can do nothing about. Notice what thought about the experience is unhelpful (i.e. either makes you feel worse or involves an action with detrimental effects).

Unhelpful thought. Example: I don't want to go to work:

_____

_____

Make that thought more helpful with the following statements: "It is true that" Unhelpful thought, Example: I don't want to go to work and, at the same time "positive that is also true". Example: I love getting paychecks

_____

_____

"Given that" Unhelpful thought. Example: I don't want to go to work:

_____

_____

Unhelpful thought, "What do I want to do with this day, situation, etc." Focus on how happy it makes me to see the check deposited into my bank account and know that I'm working towards that: Unhelpful thought: Example: I don't want to go to work

_____

_____

*Do one of the following five-minute meditations and then record whatever you experience.

1) Imagine how someone who is "calm and in control" would act in the same situation.

2) Get in touch with every aspect of the situation that is going favorably and express appreciation, in your mind, to whatever you feel to be responsible for this. (e.g. I appreciate my savings are growing, thanks to my work). This will help to keep you motivated through inevitable frustrations.

_____

_____

_____

_____

_____

15. Define and Work Towards Goals

One way to manage impulses is to have a goal. By defining and working towards a goal, you can achieve what you desire in the long term, regardless of how many times you are sidetracked along the way. Research shows people who work towards defined goals are happier than those who do not. This is due to the way the brain engages in the process of getting to the goal, more than the achievement of the goal itself.

Think of something you want to learn, accomplish, or do; it should be something you can begin within the next month. Maybe you've always wanted to learn another language, or a dance style; perhaps you want to create a scrapbook or write a book. Create one goal for this month, then lay out the steps you will take towards achieving it.

Unlike a business plan or something you *should* do, this goal is something you want to do just because it interests you. It doesn't matter how much is accomplished by the end of the month. The point of the exercise is to observe the process to see whether setting goals and working towards them decreases the negative consequences of impulsivity and increases your happiness.

Let's say you chose to begin to learn Japanese. (Learning a language is a good choice because there is always something more that can be achieved.) Using a calendar, break your goal for the month into smaller steps. Maybe you will learn a certain number of words each day, attend a certain number of classes over the month, do something each week, etc. Depending on what feels right to you, create steps and set target dates for accomplishing the steps during the month. Now, start working towards the goal, and notice how you feel during the various parts of the process. Remember it may be easier and feel more pleasurable to watch TV or do nothing, but happiness will come from engaging your brain towards achieving something.

Take Action

Choose a goal that is important to you, and about which you will feel good achieving. Write steps you can take towards this goal, and do them for the remainder of the month. Remember the most important part of this exercise is to observe the process.

My goal is:

_____

_____

_____

To work towards this goal, I will:

_____

_____

_____

What I observed about this process was (e.g. how motivated I stayed, how important it felt, the energy I sustained towards reaching it):

Congratulations on having set a goal and taken steps toward achieving it.

References

Berridge, K.C., & Robinson, T.E. (2008). What is the role of dopamine in reward: Hedonic impact, reward learning, or incentive salience? *Brain Research Reviews, 309–369*

Energizer (1994). Star Wars Energizer Bunny commercial. YouTube. Retrieved January 2012 from http://www.youtube.com/watch?v=QxafIhYFOr0.

Hallowell, E. (2005, January). Overloaded Circuits: Why Smart People Underperform. *Harvard Business Review*

Healy, J. (1998, May). Understanding TV's Effects on the Developing Brain. *American Academy of Pediatrics, AAP News.*

Human multitasking (n.d.). Wikipedia. Retrieved from http://en.wikipedia.org/wiki/Human_multitasking.

Karat, C.M., Halverson, C., Horn, D., & Karat, J. (1999). Patterns of entry and correction in large vocabulary continuous speech recognition systems. *CHI 99 Conference Proceedings, 568–575.*

Lieberman, M. D., Eisengerger, N. I., Crockett, M. J., Tom, S. M., Pfeifer, J. H., & Way, B. M., (2007). Putting feelings into words: Affect labeling disrupts amygdala activity in response to affective stimuli. *Psychological Science, 5,* 421-428.

Science Daily. (2006, July 26). Multi-tasking Adversely Affects Brain's Learning. Retrieved from http://www.sciencedaily.com

Radiological Society of North America. (2006). Violent Video Games Leave Teenagers Emotionally Aroused. *Science Daily,* retrieved from http://www.sciencedaily.com

Ritter, M. (2008) Scientists concerned about effect of technology on brain. *Associated Press,* December 3, 2008.

Small, G, MD.(2009, May 1). Don't let computer use harm your brain. *Bottom Line/Health*

Swink, D. (2010, April 14). Put that iPhone down, I'm talking to you. *Psychology Today*

Stahl, S. (2008). *Stahl's Essential Psychopharmacology*, Cambridge University Press, 3rd Edition, March 17, 2008.

Other Resources

ONLINE

ADD Resources
www.addresources.org
Information and support to help people with ADHD achieve their full
potential

ADDitude Magazine
www.additudemag.com
Magazine for people with ADHD

ADDvance Online
www.addvance.com
Online resource for women and girls with ADHD

ADD Warehouse
www.addwarehouse.com
Collection of ADHD-related books, videos, training programs, games, professional texts and assessment products

Attention Deficit Disorder Association
www.add.org
Provides information, resources and networking opportunities to help adults
with ADHD lead better lives

Centers for Disease Control
www.cdc.gov/ncbddd/adhd
A trusted source for facts and general information about ADHD

Children and Adults with Attention Deficit/ Hyperactivity Disorder
www.CHADD.org
Non-profit, membership organization that provides resources, local groups,
education, advocacy and support for those with ADHD

National Resource Center on ADHD
www.help4adhd.org
Funded by the CDC, science-based information about ADHD and ADD

BOOKS

ADD in the Workplace: Choices, Changes and Challenges
Kathleen G. Nadeau Ph.D

ADD on the Job: Making Your ADD Work For You
Lynn Weiss, Ph.D

ADD & Romance
Jonathan Scott Halverstadt, MS

*Driven to Distraction: Recognizing and Coping with Attention Deficit
Disorder from Childhood through Adulthood*
Edward M. Hallowell, MD and John J. Ratey, MD

Feeling Good
David Burns, MD

The Disorganized Mind
Nancy A. Ratey, M.Ed

About the Author

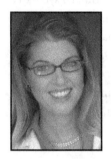

Born in the Midwest, **Dr. Alicia Ruelaz Maher** completed college and medical school in only six years, at the University of Missouri-Kansas City, School of Medicine. In the midst of her schooling, she took a year to travel around the world, studying medicine in various cultures. She then came to Los Angeles where she completed a psychiatry residency at Harbor-UCLA Medical Center and a fellowship in Mind-Body, or Psychosomatic Medicine, through UCLA. She then went on to become the Associate Director of the Psychiatric Consultation Service of Cedars-Sinai Medical Center and Associate Professor of Psychiatry at UCLA.

Through over 15 years of studying, practicing and teaching in academic medicine, living yoga in yearly ashram retreats, and observing medical care during travel to more than 30 countries, Dr. Maher has developed a "Spiritual Neuroscience" that integrates alternative and western medicine, spirituality and neuroscience for innovation in current medical practice. For Dr. Maher, spirituality is defined as whatever helps someone to be a better version of themselves and incorporates all that an individual brings to their path, as they become who they desire to be. She views our mental and physical challenges as important steps in a person's unique journey. By using tools she's developed from the latest neuroscience research, she guides clients in understanding and utilizing their brains more effectively.

Known to 'meet patients where they are' Dr. Maher works with clients to discover their unique optimum mental wellness. She then offers a wide array of resources including medication, psychotherapy, alternative therapies, Eastern practices and other modalities, allowing the client to choose what feels right to them at that moment. For those facing medical issues, she is available to work closely with other practitioners in order to facilitate a team approach to care that recognizes the interplay between the mind and body.

Qualified to treat the full spectrum of mental health conditions, Dr. Maher has particular interest in treating individuals through their medical conditions, life transitions, weight management and Attention Deficit Disorder (ADD and ADHD).

Dr. Maher has been active in teaching the next generation of doctors of USC and UCSF, UCLA medical school and has trained Cedars-Sinai Psychiatry residents. She has lectured to thousands of professionals and individuals on a wide variety of mental health and wellness topics. She has written articles for medical journals including the *Journal of American Medical Association* (JAMA), *Medscape, Psychiatric Times, Journal of General Internal Medicine, The International Association for Cognitive Behavioral Therapy* and several others. In addition to her medical practice in Southern California, Dr. Maher does healthcare research through the RAND Corporation.